Notes On... Nursing Leadership

Notes On… Nursing Leadership

Dr. Alison H. James
Dr. David Stanley

WILEY Blackwell

Registered Offices

John Wiley & Sons, Inc., 111 River Street, Hoboken, NJ 07030, USA

John Wiley & Sons Ltd, The Atrium, Southern Gate, Chichester, West Sussex, PO19 8SQ, UK

For details of our global editorial offices, customer services, and more information about Wiley products visit us at www.wiley.com.

Wiley also publishes its books in a variety of electronic formats and by print-on-demand. Some content that appears in standard print versions of this book may not be available in other formats.

Library of Congress Cataloging-in-Publication Data applied for:

Paperback ISBN: 9781394230198

Cover design: Wiley

Set in 9.5/12.5pt STIXTwoText by Straive, Pondicherry, India

Printed and bound by CPI Group (UK) Ltd, Croydon, CR0 4YY

C9781394230198_010224

Contents

Preface

The landscape of healthcare provision across the world has changed in the past few years. An increased dependence on technology, growing financial pressure on the world's health services, the potential impact of AI, an ongoing shortage of qualified nursing and other health professional staff, the global pandemic, political turmoil and a host of other regional and local pressures has meant the act of providing and leading care in the healthcare domain or health service has come under growing pressure. In addition, the path towards becoming a nurse or health professional has changed, with unprecedented clinical challenges and changes in the way students learn. The provision of methods and content of education has required a rapid response as a result and the effectiveness of this is hugely important for the future of the healthcare workforce. The global pandemic has exposed weaknesses in health services around the world, but it has also emphasised the commitment, care and courage health professionals have been able to bring to their roles each day and in a multitude of clinical environments.

Today's nursing and health professional students are leaders for tomorrow's healthcare, and this book outlines the key aspects of leadership and what leadership means for today's health professionals facing sustained and ongoing change and clinical challenges. Nurses and other health professionals are expected to employ a solid knowledge base, sound clinical skills and think critically and to do so with a firm grasp of what it means to lead and how leadership is applied in the health service. However, this too is coming under pressure from the same forces mentioned above with the additional challenges of burnout, compassion fatigue, bullying and a seeming host of more hostile detractors of the importance of professionalism. Yet those who embrace the challenges of being a healthcare professional do so with strength of belief in their worth and value to communities and society, and this is the potency from which great leadership evolves.

This text *Notes On. . . Nursing Leadership* is written to provide an outline or overview of what it means to be a nurse leader in the health service, with a focus on the perspective of a clinical nurse. Its aim is to help nurses and health professionals understand how concepts, skills and context within nursing leadership is applied and how effective nurse leadership can, or might, be used to enhance individual development, clinical practice and the overall health services and patient care.

Acknowledgements

This book would not have been possible without the support of a wide host of people including the team at Wiley-Blackwell including Tom Marriott, Christabel Daniel Raj, Naveen Kumaran, and Swetha Kodimari, who have provided excellent and detailed support for the book's production. Our writing colleagues, Clare Bennett and Dominic Roche, have been wonderful in joining this project and participating with writing contributions and practical advice and feedback.

In addition, thank you to our academic colleagues from around the world, who have offered encouragement and support especially those at Cardiff University.

About the Authors

ALISON H. JAMES DAHP, MA, PGCE, BA, DIP HE, RGN, BA, SFHEA

Alison began her nursing career in 1986 qualifying as a Registered Nurse and working in neurosciences for her formative years. Having previously completed a BA in Humanities, Alison then completed a Diploma in Critical Care and BA in Healthcare Studies before moving into clinical research nursing. Completing an MA in Healthcare Law and Ethics, Alison then worked as a Knowledge Transfer Consultant in health and social care for several years and returned to Wales in 2014 as an academic in adult nursing at Cardiff University where she completed her Doctorate in Advanced Healthcare Practice. This has enabled Alison to focus on her research and scholarship in healthcare leadership and she is currently a Reader in the School of Healthcare Sciences where she continues to teach and research her area of interest, publishing and speaking internationally. Having previously co-authored *Clinical Leadership in Nursing and Healthcare* with David Stanley and Clare Bennett, Alison continues to contribute to evidence and scholarship in this area.

DAVID STANLEY NursD, MSC HS, BA NG, DIP HE (NURSING), EX-RN, EX-RM, TF, GERONTIC CERT, GRAD CERT HPE

David began his nursing career in the days when nurses wore huge belt buckles and funny hats. He 'trained' as a Registered Nurse and Midwife in South Australia and worked through his formative career in several hospitals and clinical environments in Australia. In 1993, he completed a Bachelor of Nursing at Flinders University, Adelaide, and, after a number of years of volunteer work in Africa, he moved to the United Kingdom and worked as the Coordinator of Children's Services and as a Nurse Practitioner. He completed a Master of Health Science degree at Birmingham University. For a short time, he worked in Central Australia for Remote Health Services before returning to the United Kingdom to complete his nursing doctorate, researching clinical leadership. This resulted in the development of a new values-based leadership theory: *Congruent Leadership*. He continued to research in the areas of clinical leadership, men in nursing and the role of the media in nursing while contributing to teaching roles at several Australian Universities. He has recently retired from nursing and is focused on writing poetry and fiction.

About the Notes On... Series

Florence Nightingale wrote two health focused books, *"Notes on Nursing"* and *"Notes on Hospitals"*; however, this series of short books inspired by her use of the *"Notes on"* title is developed to address a range of nursing and health professional specific topics in brief or note form. Each book in the series offers a comprehensive overview of information on a wide range of topics for nurses, midwives and other health professionals. It is hoped the books will be especially useful for health professional students in a number of professions with the books providing key, relevant, concise, information in an accessible way. *Notes On... Leadership in Nursing* is the second book in the series.

> For us who nurse, our nursing is a thing, which, unless in it we are making progress every year, every month, every week, take my word for it we are going back. The more experience we gain, the more progress we can make.
>
> Florence Nightingale (https://www.azquotes.com/quote/614045)

1

Introduction

1.1 About This Book

In 1999, Colleen Wedderburn Tate (1999, p. 3) said, *"Some healthcare staff are no longer working for patients, but are more motivated by pronouncements from government ministers, exposes in the media, and the latest scandal about misuse of public money."* As we begin this dialog about nursing leadership, we wonder if anything has changed. After decades of talking about, writing about and searching for what we mean by nurse leaders, has anything really changed in practice, at the bedside or in the involvement of nurses at the wider decision-making table? We propose that nurses, more than any other healthcare employee group, need leaders, need to gain a deep understanding of leadership and need to be leaders for the profession. Because without a clear understanding of what leadership means, how it is recognised and how it is practiced, nursing and patient care will be poorer. It is in an effort to redress this shortfall that this book is written.

We believe that since Wedderburn Tate's (1999) statement above, nurses continue to have only superficial influence over healthcare resource decisions. While managers, healthcare service administrators, many medical practitioners and their teams still see themselves as "all powerful" in terms of their decisions and leadership of nurses and some other health professionals. Thousands of nurses graduate and are employed every year, only to leave their chosen profession the following year or the one after. This is because they become frustrated by their lack of influence or power over the work they do, the contribution they could potentially

Notes On... Nursing Leadership, First Edition. Alison H. James and David Stanley.
© 2024 John Wiley & Sons Ltd. Published 2024 by John Wiley & Sons Ltd.

make or their inability to contribute to or influence decisions. They become frustrated that they can't provide the level of care they believe their clients/patients deserve. In addition, nurses often see their great ideas or projects relegated to lower priorities or ignored altogether by aloof hospital administrations and managers who (it should be acknowledged) are also under great pressure to deliver an effective health service with diminishing resources.

However, there is another issue with nurses and leadership. Nurses have been almost conditioned to see others (managers/doctors) as their leaders. When undertaking a number of studies exploring perceptions of clinical nurse leadership between 2001 and 2017 (Stanley et al. 2023), hundreds of clinical-level nurses were approached and asked to identify colleagues they saw as clinical leaders. The most common response was, "*What, nurses as leaders–no, don't you want to talk to my manager?*". Wedderburn Tate (1999) confirmed this, saying, "*nurses who are successful leaders do not recognise themselves as such*" and it seems nurses have not been taught that their leadership potential is in their hands. Reassuringly, some respondents in Stanley's studies (Stanley et al. 2012, 2014, 2017; Stanley 2019; Stanley and Stanley 2019) were able to point to highly skilled, effective and influential clinical-level nurses who displayed and practiced leadership as part of their clinical role. After decades of discussion and training about leadership in nursing, the majority of clinically focused nurses still fail to grasp the value of leadership to their practice and their responsibilities as leaders in the health service. When exploring perceptions of leadership with student nurses, James (2020) and James et al. (2022) found that student nurses rarely saw themselves as leaders then or in the future, and many felt unprepared to take on the concept of leadership. Although in the United Kingdom (UK) nurses are expected to demonstrate leadership at the point of registration, there remains a disparate approach to leadership education and preparation (James 2023). While the nursing curriculum remains full of clinical skill competencies and nurses take on more and more of these, leadership seems to be advertised as something one can pick up with a quick course. It is our opinion that leadership requires much further consideration and thought from early within the development of a nurse, application of critique to traditional theoretical positions and ownership by nursing as a profession (James et al. 2023).

It is our conclusion that nursing leadership is essential, not just to pay lip service to the nursing profession and bolster its ego or place in the scheme of the health service but to make a genuine contribution to improving patient care and making the health service more robust and responsive to client/patient needs (James et al. 2023). This book sets out to offer a clear and straightforward perspective on what nursing leadership means and how it can be recognised and applied in practice.

The book is aimed at undergraduate nurses as a useful resource and may be of use to a range of qualified and practicing nurses who wish to review their insights into nurse leadership. It aims to inspire and support nurses in both understanding and developing their approach to leadership in nursing. It also aims to serve as a useful resource for nurses who are more advanced in their careers and who are interested in developing their leadership skills and broadening their awareness or leadership potential as nurse leaders. It is a contemporary introductory text that links current key debates and thinking in leadership as it applies to nursing practice.

Chapter 1 sets out the importance of leadership in nursing and why leadership is important in nursing now. It describes how the book is structured as well as considering the difference between leadership and management. Chapter 2 begins with an oversight of definitions of leadership, nursing leadership and an exploration of several leadership theories. Chapter 3 explores the attributes seen as vital for effective nurse leadership to prevail. This is presented as hard and soft skills and attributes and it goes on to explore why these skills are vital for nurse leaders to be successful. Chapter 4 outlines the importance of an understanding of self-care for leaders to be successful and remain vital. Chapter 5 offers an outline of the role of nurse leaders in driving innovation and change in the health service. Chapter 6 provides an overview of the relationship between leadership and teams, suggesting that nurse leaders need to understand how teams function and recognise their place when helping teams work. Chapter 7 takes the relationship of the leader to others further by exploring the significance of "networking" as a skill in the "toolbox" of effective nurse leadership. Chapter 8 looks at the central place of values for nurse leaders to be their best selves. Chapter 9 deals with the challenges nurse leaders face in the application of leadership, and Chapter 10 considers the flip side of leadership, followership, and how this can impact on the effectiveness of nurse leaders. Throughout the book, the value of applying nursing leadership is outlined, and the component parts of leadership are expressed.

1.2   Leadership and Management are Different!

Leadership and management are equally important, interdependent and inter related; however, they are also different and distinct, serving different purposes and requiring different skills (St George 2012; West et al. 2015; Gumbo 2017; Leech 2019; Nene et al. 2020; Stanley et al. 2023). In the health service, leadership and management are frequently seen as one all-encompassing thing (Stanley et al. 2023). However, Wood (2021, p. 284) suggests that *"Working out who leads and who manages is difficult, with the added anomaly that not all managers are leaders, and some people who lead work in management positions."* This has the potential to lead to role ambiguity (Stanley 2006; Cutcliffe and Cleary 2015; Nene et al. 2020), and conflict can occur when clinicians take on management roles without appropriate training, support or instruction (Nene et al. 2020; Stanley et al. 2023). Likewise, tensions can occur between clinical leaders and managers, when leaders feel that their efforts are hampered by management or organisational aspirations or targets (Stanley 2006; Kerridge 2013; Orvik et al. 2015; Scully 2015; Stanley 2017a, 2017b; Nene et al. 2020). Zaleznik (1977) makes the point that management and leadership positions require different types of people which may be problematic in healthcare with the tendency for role overlap (Stanley 2006; Cutcliffe and Cleary 2015; Nene et al. 2020). Kotterman (2006) argues that a well-balanced organisation requires a blend of leaders and managers to succeed, and while there are overlaps, there is clarity in the distinction when explored further. This is important if you are interested in becoming a leader and/or manager.

Reflective Activity 1.1

Before you read on … Think about someone you have worked with who you saw/see as an inspirational leader. The only restriction placed on this activity is that you must think of a clinically focused nurse or midwife. Not a manager, not a doctor, not another health professional, not a relative or friend who is not a nurse. Think primarily of a clinically focused nurse/midwife.

Why did you think of this person?
What was it about them that made you see them as leaders?
Was it difficult to think of a nurse/midwife?
Were you drawn to think of others, of doctors, managers or other senior (non-clinical) nurses? If so, why?

1.3   The Difference

Delineating between management and leadership can help ensure that the most appropriate skill set is utilised to achieve the best outcomes in practice (Jones and Bennett 2018). Moreover, Kotter (1990a) and Bass (2010) feel that using the terms interchangeably is misleading, adding that management and leadership are not synonymous, with Bennis (1989) recognising that leaders and managers have different ways of seeing the world.

1.3.1   Management

Managerial activities are essential to the smooth running of an organisation and the attainment of care standards and targets (see an example in Box 1.1). Good managers bring order and consistency, which can ensure that key dimensions such as quality are maintained. Katz's (1955) seminal work describes management as being concerned with directing a group or organisation with a focus on task orientation, staff

---

Box 1.1   An Example of Management

An example of a fundamental management role is staff rostering. Whilst widely held as one of the more mundane aspects of clinical management, the skill involved in providing around-the-clock cover, that takes into account patient acuity, variability in admission patterns, regulations regarding staff breaks between and during shifts and staff availability, should not be underestimated (Adapted from Wynendaele et al. 2021).

development, conflict resolution and the maintenance of ethics and discipline. Kotterman (2006) describes managers as focusing on the attainment of short-term goals, risk avoidance and standardisation to enhance efficiency, with Zaleznik (1977) adding that managers promote stability, exercise authority and are task orientated. Kotter (2001) expands this definition, claiming that management is concerned with planning, organising, budgeting, coordinating and monitoring. Managers rely on strategy, structure and systems; in other words, the operational element of organisations, requiring planning, budgeting, organising, staffing, problem-solving and controlling. Watson (1983) suggests that management roles tend to be dependent upon formal positions and attained through specific training schemes such as the NHS Graduate Management Training Scheme (NHS Graduate Management Training Scheme 2021). Management is seen as procedural and task focused, while attributes of leadership include visionary, influencing qualities. Kotter (1990a) adds that management consists primarily of three things:

- analysis
- problem-solving
- planning

1.3.2 Leadership

More is offered about leadership in the next chapter (Chapter 2); however, it is clear that leadership is about the leader's values, coping with change and/or creating disruption (Stanley et al. 2023). Leaders promote change and are people orientated, with Watson (1983) and Heinen et al. (2019) asserting that leaders use the "softer" skills of leadership such as being staff focused, being style driven, having shared goals and key clinical skills. Bryman (1986) and Goleman (1998a) add that leaders are also concerned with strategic motivation, and the Healthcare Leadership Model (NHS Leadership Academy 2021) emphasises that leadership is not necessarily related to seniority within an organisation. Clinical leaders focus on motivating and inspiring others towards common goals (Kotter 1990a) as they create a passion among others to share their vision. Leaders focus on the attainment of long-term goals; they take risks, challenge the status quo and work towards adapting to change (Nene et al. 2020). Kotter (1990a) suggests that leadership consists of:

- vision,
- values and
- communication of vision and values.

With change and innovation characterising modern healthcare, the role of healthcare/clinical leadership has become more relevant in recent years, because it is integral to initiating innovation and change (West et al. 2015; Stanley et al. 2023). Innovation and change always demand more leadership (Kotter 1990a, 1990b) because of its concern with aligning people, setting direction, motivating, inspiring, employing credibility, adopting a visionary position, anticipating change and coping with change (Jones and Bennett 2018; Stanley et al. 2023). Leaders also align their leadership with the values central to the organisational goals (West et al. 2017; Stanley et al. 2023).

1.4 The Challenges Leaders and Managers Face

Management and leadership are two different, yet complementary activities (Kotter 1990b); consequently, they present several challenges. The efficient running of any organisation requires both and recognises that management is a function that must be exercised in any organisation, while leadership is a relationship between the leader and the led that can energise an organisation (Stanley et al. 2023). It is also clear that when management and leadership functions are embodied in the same person, or within the same post, it can lead to:

- values breach (Stanley 2006),
- confusion,
- conflict (Stanley 2006) and
- diminished clinical and management effectiveness (Kippist and Fitzgerald 2009; Kerridge 2013; Cutcliffe and Cleary 2015; Veronesi et al. 2019; Nene et al. 2020).

Leadership and management are different. You cannot manage a person into battle or into the teeth of a global health emergency – they must be led.

It is also clear that within healthcare, both leadership and management are essential to ensure patient safety and inspire innovation and change and are central to improving the efficiency of clinical areas and developing sustainable improvements in the quality of patient/client care. For a genuine opportunity to develop more efficient clinical management and clearer, more effective nursing leadership, it may be time to accept that having leadership and management functions reside in one person or post is inefficient and counterproductive, both to the individual concerned and to the health service's future development and success.

Since the 1970s, numerous authors have highlighted the differences between leadership and management (Zaleznik 1977; Stanley 2006, 2017b). The health industry is constantly dealing with change, and organisations need both effective and values-focused leaders and managers (Kline 2019). Sometimes it is the manager who fulfils a leadership role, while at other times, others within the organisation lead (see Box 1.2).

To suggest that only managers can lead is an outdated concept. However, many of our healthcare organisations are built on years of hierarchical traditions, and positional roles are sometimes viewed as leadership when they are in fact more managerial in description. Leadership occurs on many levels, and effective managers will acknowledge this and utilise the skills of staff to support quality and innovation within the organisation. Maintaining the status quo requires considerable energy, and working as a manager in any health organisation demands resilience, commitment and dedication. Managers are about stability, running the organisation and keeping things on an even keel. Anderson's (2012) view is that only some managers are able to lead and engage in both stable management tasks and creative risk-taking leadership. Appointing and training people who are asked to function as

---

Box 1.2   Role Confusion

One of the key criticisms identified by the Francis Inquiry (Francis 2013) was that confusion existed because a care culture had developed where management was separated from ward-level leadership, and as a result confusion existed over who should be responsible for care. The net impact was a breakdown of communication and a loss of focus on high-quality client/patient care.

managers but with expectations that they will offer dynamic and risk-taking leadership sets them up to fail or leads them to feel insecure in their role (Vize 2015).

Recognising the difference between leadership and management will allow professional development to embrace education focused on leadership development that is based on clinical practice and not simply management principles overlaid on clinical functions. Walker (2016) argues that the increasing complexity of healthcare systems requires a different style of leadership and management. She proposes that traditional hierarchical models should be replaced by an approach whereby accountability is distributed across multiple stakeholders and that interdisciplinary collaboration is given priority (Stanley and Stanley 2018; NHS England 2023). Walker (2016) asserts that we need leaders who are able to:

- align purpose and practice,
- create and nurture networks and
- give up a degree of autonomy to foster interdependency.

Walker (2016) also argues that leaders and managers will need to reorientate health services towards wellness and quality, which will create the need for buy-in through effective engagement with stakeholders as well as inspire the workforce to want to achieve system goals through motivational communication. There is also a need for nursing to develop its own approach to leadership, using the potency of its knowledge, skills and experience to inspire future nurse leaders (James et al. 2023). This is only possible if we encourage nursing leaders to hold a values-based leadership focus, and this should be the primary focus of leadership in nursing.

1.5 Summary

This chapter has outlined that the book's focus is on nursing leadership and that leadership in nursing cannot be considered without an insight into management and why leadership and management are different. It suggests that leadership has been a difficult concept for nursing to come to grips with, yet it remains a vital element for nurses to apply and understand if they are to genuinely impact quality patient care, safety, innovation and change in their local and wider health service.

Reflective Activity 1.2

Before you read on ... Think about your idea of the difference between leadership and management. Are they the same or different things?

Can one person be both a leader and a manager?
Might this cause conflict for them or their team?
Make a list of six words that define or describe a leader and a manager.
Are there any words that you used in both list?

2

What Is This Leadership Thing?

2.1 Introduction

This chapter will explore definitions of nursing leadership and provide a brief overview of a host of leadership theories. The study of leadership and attempts to describe and understand it are not new and leadership is seen as central to all aspects of nursing (Ellis 2021). For centuries writers, philosophers, leaders and the led have explored the characteristics of "great" leaders and looked at how they came to lead and what influence they have had on their relationships with their followers, history, decisions made and even any adverse impacts of their leadership decisions. There is one simple overarching theme in all the musings on this topic: trying to describe or understand leadership is not easy or straightforward and there seems to be no one way to relate everything there is to understand about leadership.

Nursing has a troubled relationship with leadership with the origins of the profession based on a model of servitude, self-sacrifice and subservience to the medical profession, in much the same way soldiers deferred to their officers' orders and nuns bowed to the whims and demands of the male clergy who oversaw their work and practice. Leadership was not something seriously considered relevant as part of a nurse's curriculum late into the 21st century. This is changing, although it has perhaps become one of those terms too loosely applied and too little understood, and nurses still need to be encouraged to see that leadership is something more than a position or title or based on notions of hierarchy or power.

Notes On... Nursing Leadership, First Edition. Alison H. James and David Stanley.
© 2024 John Wiley & Sons Ltd. Published 2024 by John Wiley & Sons Ltd.

> **Reflective Activity 2.1**
>
> Before you read on … Reflect upon your understanding of the word "*leadership*."
> Now reflect on the words "*nurse leader*."
> Think about why nurses should be focused on the topic of leadership, and consider a nurse you recognise as a leader.

2.2 Defining Leadership

There are a plethora of definitions of leader and leadership and some even seem to contradict each other. However, many thinkers see leaders as having some sort of influence over the actions of others in order to accomplish goals (Stogdill 1948; Northouse 2007; Grossman and Valiga 2021). Leadership can also be viewed as achieving things with the support of others (Leigh and Maynard 1995) or because the leader has authority over others (Fiedler 1967; Dublin 1968). Stogdill's (1948) view is that leadership is the process of influencing people or the activities of a group to accomplish goals. This perspective brings in the concept of influence and acknowledges that people without formal power can exercise leadership. Leadership is also seen as, "*a talent that each of us has and that can be learned, developed, and nurtured. Most importantly it is not necessarily tied to a position of authority in an organisation*" (Grossman and Valiga 2021, p. 18).

> **Definition of Leadership According to the New Oxford Dictionary of English (NODE 2021)**
>
> Leadership is "*The action of leading a group of people or an organization.*" https://www.tlu.ee/~sirvir/Leadership/The%20Concept%20of%20Leadership/definitions_of_leadership.html#:~:text=Conclusion-,Definitions%20of%20Leadership,'%20(NODE%2C%202001).

Kotter (1990a, p. 40) proposes that as well as goal setting and influence, leadership is about effecting change saying, "*leadership is all about coping with change.*" Bennis and Nanus (1985, p. 3), supporting Kotter's

(1990a) suggestion, add that a leader is "*one who commits people to action, who converts followers into leaders and who converts leaders into agents of change.*" These views suggest that change is central to the application of leadership, and they support the assumption that a leader's function within an organisation is to promote and support change, rather than establish stability. Pedler et al. (2004) propose that elements of the leader's character and the context within which the leadership takes place also matter for a clear insight of leadership to evolve.

More recently, leadership has been viewed as attending to the meanings and values of the group rather than just the authority, function, challenges and traits of the leader. Covey (1992) describes what he called "*principle-centred leadership*" and Pondy (1978) similarly proposed that leadership is the ability to make activities meaningful and not necessarily to change behaviour, giving others a sense that what they are doing is meaningful, describing this as the core of leadership. Therefore, the act of leading is about making the meaning of an activity explicit. "*Unlike the supposed individualistic leadership of the past, now leadership is influenced by the impact of the immediate and surrounding context . . .*" (Kakabadse and Kakabadse 1999, p. 2). The suggestion here is that (the) organisational context(s) provides the parameters within which current leadership is contained. From this perspective it can be argued that the task of the leader is to interpret and clarify the context and thus provide a platform for communicating meaning within the organisation's activity.

As a result, leadership becomes more about selecting, synthesising and articulating an appropriate vision for the follower (Bennis et al. 1995). Greenfield (1986) takes this concept of vision further by implying that rather than just clarifying the meaning or making the activity meaningful, leadership is about setting the meaning, describing leadership as "*a wilful act where one person attempts to construct the social world for others . . . leaders will try to commit others to the values that they themselves believe are good and that organizations* (sic) *are built on the unification of people around values*" (Greenfield 1986, p. 166).

Day et al. (2000), like Greenfield (1986), support the notion that the leader is the one who is responsible for "*establishing core characteristics*" (Bell and Ritchie 1999, p. 24), for committing others to their values and setting the overall organisational aims. If we consider these carefully, the importance of leadership on organisational cultures becomes clear.

Leaders set the tone, set the boundaries and possibilities, and establish what is acceptable and what is not within an organisation or team.

There are a wide variety of definitions and perspectives of leadership and leadership is rightly seen as a complex process having multiple dimensions (Northouse 2007; Jones and Bennett 2018). Still, it is clear that no one definition can be considered wholly right or wrong. Varied perspectives and definitions, and perhaps an eclectic view of leadership, may prove most beneficial with Duke (1986, p. 10) suggesting that *"leadership seems to be a gestalt phenomenon; greater than the sum of its parts."* This said, the definition below is offered as a way of summarising how leadership may be understood within the context of leadership in nursing. Nursing leadership is about *unifying people around core values and then constructing the social world around those values, inspiring innovation and helping people get through change.*

2.3 Definition of Nurse Leadership

Marie Morganelli Bell (2021) defined nurse leadership as *"the ability to inspire, influence and motivate health care professionals as they work together to achieve their goals"* (https://www.snhu.edu/about-us/newsroom/health/what-is-nurse-leadership#:~:text=Nurse%20leadership%20is%20the%20ability,Dr.), while Cline et al. (2022) are of the view that the term *"nurse leadership"* is still defined in multiple ways. As such, they set out to present a new definition of *"nurse leader"* that can be adopted by all nurse professionals across practice continuums and globally. Cline et al. (2022, p. 383) suggested that the word *"nurse"* implied leadership and that nurse leadership should be defined by a set of actions such as *"leading with integrity, compassion, and humility"* and that because nursing was grounded in *"empathetic action"* and a *"commitment to human dignity,"* because nurses use *"evidence, inspired innovation"* and were *"courageous,"* they should be considered leaders. Their paper offers a word cloud to help explain the term nurse leader, but a clear definitive definition is still lacking and the term remains ill defined. However, the following definition of nursing leadership is offered here:

> *Nurse leaders are able to lead with their values about care and compassion to the fore to inspire, influence and motivate nurse colleagues and other healthcare professionals as they work*

collaboratively towards the promotion of safe, effective person-centred healthcare and positive, productive collegial relationships.

2.4 Theories of Leadership

There is a plethora of leadership theories, many have emerged from business and other disciplines and others are more focused and developed from evidence within nursing and healthcare. Clark and Thompson (2022) are sceptical of what they term the "leadership illusion" that pervades modern nursing; so while theories can provide background and ideas, it is important to also consider with criticality what theory can be best applied and align to nursing. The main ones and those most relevant for nursing are outlined below.

2.4.1 The Great Man Theory

Galton (1869), Man (2010) and Khan et al. (2016) suggested that leadership was a matter of birth, or was assigned by divine decree, with Bennis and Nanus (1985, p. 5) adding that *"those of the right breed could lead."* Implying that leaders came from great families and that their leadership potential (and right) was passed down through the male line in succession and given by divine power. This theory has been debunked as it is clear that leaders can come from any level of society and be of any gender (Grossman and Valiga 2021; Stanley et al., 2023).

2.4.2 The Heroic Leader

Heroic leadership is sometimes called *"charismatic leadership"* (Khan et al. 2016) and as Lowney (2003) suggests rests on four principles: self-awareness, ingenuity, love and heroism. However, heroic leaders are often driven by goal scoring, and they lead alone, setting the tone for others to follow, by virtue of their courageous actions.

2.4.3 The Big Bang Theory

This theory appeared in the wake of the calamitous events of the early 20th century, with old ideas of leadership failing and leaders rising from the great events of the time, to lead without formal training, status or rank. Bennis and Nanus (1985, p. 5) suggested that *"great events made leaders of otherwise ordinary people."* This theory proposes that it is circumstances or events that reveal the leader, ignoring any previous experience or hard work the leaders may have undertaken to be prepared to take on the leadership role (Stanley et al. 2023).

2.4.4 Trait Theory

This theory rests on the assumption that the individual leader is more significant than the situation the leader is in. As such, leaders can be recognised by distinguishing features or characteristics, common to all leaders (Khan et al. 2016; Swanwick and McKimm 2017). Many researchers and writers have sought over the past century to identify what these might be (Stogdill 1948, 1974; Mann 1959; Kirkpatrick and Locke 1991; Smith 1999; Grossman and Valiga 2021) and no clear definitive list is evident. As well as failing to identify specific attributes, the theory neglects the impact of the leadership situation within which the leaders operate (Northouse 2007) or the leader's personality when leadership is called for (Mann 1959).

2.4.5 Style Theory

These theories explore how leaders behave with leaders being described as **Democratic, Paternalistic, Lasses-faire, Autocratic** and/or **Dictatorial** (Handy 1999; Lett 2002; Northouse 2007). These words are used to describe the "style" of the leader and to offer a view on the benefits or drawbacks of the leader's approach to their followers and leadership responsibilities. These words are also used to describe approaches to management and give a simple overview of how the leader/manager is perceived or behaves. There are other words used to describe leadership styles, which are **Coaching, Directing, Delegating, Supporting, Charismatic, Participatory, Visionary, Pacesetting, Affirmative, Commanding, the Quiet Leader**. The descriptive words are useful but only on a superficial level and apart from offering an insight into the leader's general style, little else about their values or beliefs or leadership preferences is clear. Some of the styles can be related to other leadership theories, although the styles alone offer only limited insights into developing a leadership profile.

2.4.6 Situational or Contingency Theory

Fiedler (1967) proposed the "situational" or "contingency theory" of leadership that explored why some leaders are successful in certain situations and not in others. Fiedler (1967), Tannenbaum and Schmidt (1958), Vroom and Yetton (1973), House and Mitchell (1974) and Hersey and Blanchard (1988) believed that leadership effectiveness was dependent on the relationship between the leader's task at hand, the leader's interpersonal skills and the favourability of the work situation. Fiedler (1967) found that leaders were more effective if the situation they were trying to function within was more favourable to them or, surprisingly, less favourable. The three factors relate to:

- the degree of trust and respect that the followers have for the leader,
- the clarity of the objectives to be achieved and
- the degree of power in terms of whether the leader could reward or punish the followers or if the leader had clear organisational backing (Handy 1999, pp. 103–105).

From Fiedler's perspective, the key to understanding leadership is to be able to adapt the leadership approach to complement the issue being faced or to determine the appropriate action based on the people involved and the prevailing situation (Adair 1998). Central to Fiedler's (1967) work was the ability to analyse how the leader could use power and influence without losing respect and credibility with the subordinate group. Criticism of Fiedler's (1967) situational–contingency theory is that leadership is more complicated than the relationship between these three central factors (Adair 1998; Handy 1999) and that the theory is heavily management focused and may be more useful in terms of understanding human resource management, improving employee and workforce production, and support for the development of managers.

2.4.7 Transformational Leadership Theory

Transformational leadership was developed to understand the distinction between leadership and management and to address the question of why some leaders can inspire their followers even when the situation is less than ideal (Northouse 2007). Bass (1985) suggested that transformational leadership is about motivating followers to do more than expected by providing an idealised influence, inspirational motivation and vision. Transformational leadership is also strongly associated with the qualitative studies of Bennis and Nanus (1985) who suggested that transformational leadership connects the process of attending to the needs of the followers, so that the interaction of each raised the motivation and energy of the other and that it is about challenging the status quo, creating a vision and sharing that vision. As such, transformational leaders are able to establish and gain support for their vision while being consistently and persistently driven towards maintaining momentum and empowering others (Kakabadse and Kakabadse 1999; Swanwick and McKimm 2017).

Bennis and Nanus (1985) identified four themes pivotal to effective transformational leadership:

- *Vision*, or the ability to have a dream and to actually deliver on it.
- *Communication*, or the ability to articulate the vision so that it steals into the imagination and the minds of the followers.
- *Trust*, or the ability of the followers to feel that their leader is consistent, has integrity and can be relied on.
- *Self-knowledge (self-knowing)*, or what Bennis and Nanus (1985, p. 57) described as the ability to "know their worth . . . trust themselves without letting their ego or image get in the way."

The transformational leader's role is to communicate a vision that gives meaning to the work of others and, crucially, to reconstruct the context in which people work, removing the old and replacing it with the new. Therefore, the transformational leader need not be associated with status or power and is seen as being appropriate at all levels of an organisation. Lavoie-Tremblay et al. (2015) suggested that supportive leadership practice is able to impact upon increasing retention and improving patient care, while Weng et al. (2015) in a substantial Taiwanese research study suggested that there is a significant correlation between transformational leadership and innovation within the nursing workforce.

2.4.8 Transactional Leadership Theory

Transactional leadership is the flip side of transformational leadership with Burns (1978) describing it as the antithesis of transformational leadership, with transactional leadership existing where there is an exchange relationship between leader and followers (Jones and Bennett 2018). The role of the transactional leader is to focus on the purpose of the organisation and to assist people to recognise what needs to be done in order to reach a desired outcome through a reward/punishment motivator (Jones and Bennett 2018). Kakabadse and Kakabadse (1999) describe transactional leadership as the skill and ability required to deal with the mundane, operational and day-to-day transactions of organisational life sometimes calling this type of leadership "*transactional management*." Transactional leaders, in order to lead, need to effectively manage the more routine tasks, partly in order to retain their credibility but also to keep the organisation on track (Burns 1978).

2.4.9 Authentic/Breakthrough Leadership

"*Authentic leadership*" (Bhindi and Duignan 1997; George 2003; Avolio and Gardner 2005; Cantwell 2015) and "*breakthrough leadership*" (Sarros and Butchatsky 1996) are more recent leadership theories. The "*breakthrough*" leader and "*authentic*" leader respect and listen to others and are guided by their passion and meaning, purpose and values (Sarros and Butchatsky 1996; Bhindi and Duignan 1997; George 2003; Avolio and Gardner 2005; Cantwell 2015). Both these perspectives of leadership point towards an approach where leaders are thought to be true to their own values and beliefs, and the leader's credibility rests on their integrity and ability to be seen as a role model, because of these values and beliefs. Wong and Cummings (2009) suggest that authentic leadership is a suitable theory for aligning future nursing leadership practice. As such, authentic leadership can be described as the "glue" used to hold a healthy work environment together (Shirley 2006) with leaders being encouraged to engage with employees and promote positive behaviours.

2.4.10 Servant Leadership Theory

In keeping with some of the key elements of authentic leadership, "*servant leadership*" focuses on the leader's stewardship role and encourages leaders to "*serve*" others while staying in tune with the organisation's goals and values (Swanwick and McKimm 2017; Jones and Bennett 2018).

The concept of servant leadership was coined and defined by Robert Greenleaf (1977), who stated that servant leaders rely less on hierarchical position and more on collaboration, trust, empathy and the use of ethical power.

Servant leadership is described as suited to service-orientated organisations with benefits for supporting, valuing and developing people. Anderson (2003), Kerfoot (2004), Swearingen and Liberman (2004), Campbell and Rudisill (2005), Peete (2005), Robinson (2006), Thorne (2006), Walker (2006), Swanwick and McKimm (2017) and Jones and Bennett (2018) all emphasise the relevance of servant leadership as a model to support the development of nursing and healthcare leadership as it has a focus on promoting user involvement and on patients as the foundation of the health service, and because it is valued as a model to support staff and influence current staff retention issues (Swearingen and Liberman 2004). Hanse et al. (2016) were able to show that nurse managers who demonstrated servant leadership had stronger exchange relationships in terms of empowerment, humility and stewardship with followers. Servant leadership is also valued because according to Spears (1995) its key principles are:

- listening,
- conceptualisation,
- empathy,
- foresight,
- healing,
- stewardship,
- awareness,
- commitment to the growth of people,
- persuasion and
- building community.

Eicher-Catt (2005) believes that servant leadership is a myth and unworkable in the real world as it fails to live up to its promise of being gender-neutral and, in fact, because the paradoxical language and apposition of "*servant*" and "*leader*" accentuates gender bias, it ends up supporting androcentric patriarchal norms. There is also an argument put forward by Avolio and Gardner (2005) that servant leadership has not been developed from an empirical base and is therefore purely theoretical.

Reflective Activity 2.2

Before you read on ... Reflect upon the ward, unit, clinic or clinical area you work in. What management/leadership style does the ward manager, clinical manager or therapy team leader (or whatever they are called) adopt?
Discuss this (tactfully) with them. What style do they feel they have adopted?
Are you both in agreement?

2.4.11   Shared/Collaborative Leadership

Shared or collaborative leadership is a new concept (Pearce and Conger 2003). It occurs when two or more team members engage or participate in the act of leadership in an effort to maximise team effectiveness (Bergman et al. 2012) with Carson et al. (2007) proposing that shared leadership is based on a shared purpose, social support and a shared voice for the team. Towler (2019) suggests that it is important to distinguish shared leadership from team leadership because shared leadership describes how team members influence each other and share responsibility for tasks, rather than the concept of a team being led by a specific leader. Shared or collaborative leadership is sometimes called distributed leadership with all three having the same basic components of leadership (Northouse 2007).

2.4.12   Compassionate Leadership

Compassionate leadership is a relatively new leadership concept. West (2021) describes compassionate leadership as a strategy based on the core human value of compassion, showing that by sustaining compassion in health and social care, health professionals can cultivate wisdom, humanity, presence and high-quality care delivery in health and care services. The King's Fund (2017) also suggest that compassionate leadership can have many positive outcomes, at all levels of the health sector. It proposed that staff are more likely to find new and improved ways of doing things if they feel they are listened to, valued and supported as this provides a sense of psychological safety.

It was proposed that compassionate leadership gave NHS staff autonomy in their work, a shared sense of responsibility and a flatter hierarchical approach. In addition, compassionate leadership was thought to promote greater diversity, inclusion, creativity and innovation at all levels of an organisation. It also proposed that a compassionate approach to leadership might be a powerful facilitator for problem-solving within the health service. Compassion is described as the quality of having positive intentions and real concern for others so that compassionate leaders create stronger connections between people, improving collaboration, raising levels of trust and enhancing loyalty.

2.4.13   Congruent Leadership

The theory of "*congruent leadership*" developed from the results of research specifically designed to explore clinical nurse leadership from the perspective of several health professional disciplines between 2000 and 2017. The results of the studies proposed a new leadership theory called *congruent leadership* (Stanley 2008, 2019; Stanley et al. 2023). Congruent leadership explains leadership predominantly located in the clinical area, at the bedside, in the clinic, for the paramedic at the roadside and across all healthcare-related disciplines. The theory suggests that leaders demonstrate a match (congruence) between the leader's values and beliefs, and their actions, with followers identifying the leader's values and beliefs and feeling an affinity with them, they willingly follow. Research results indicated that clinically focused nurses and a range of health professionals who have moved decisively and clearly in the direction of their core values and beliefs can be seen expressing congruent leadership (Coventry and Russell 2021).

When acting out or role modelling their values and beliefs (even subconsciously), something was happening in their relationships with their clients, patients or colleagues that gave a clear signal about what they believed or what their values were. This linked congruent leadership with the expression of emotional intelligence and values-based relationship building and caring/compassionate engagement. Congruent leaders are described as being visible in practice, role models for the behaviour they espoused and communicating well. They were able to make effective decisions, were empowered, were compassionate and caring and could motivate others and, because their actions were evident or matched their values and beliefs, they were seen as passionate and committed leaders. This was rarely because they were visionaries, in powerful positions or wielded great authority, it was often simply because they put their core values into action for others to see and follow.

2.4.14 Conscious Leadership

Crane and Ward (2016) proposed support for the application of "conscious leadership" specifically in the application of self-care (see Chapter 4). They described a conscious leader as one who practices in the present moment and is skilled in creating environments where people can thrive. Leading this way requires the leader to focus on both the nurse (employee) and the systems that support nursing practice. Nurses are helped to choose self-care and self-healing practices and the conscious leader aims to provide a supportive work environment while demonstrating effective emotional intelligence. Crane and Ward (2016) suggest the following strategies that conscious leaders could employ:

- Posting beautiful pictures around the department/ward.
- Alerting people each shift-change, team meeting or huddle that someone has accomplished self-care or self-healing.
- Referencing self-care and self-nurturing daily and in appropriate conversations.
- Rewarding self-care and self-healing behaviours (they do not say how).

Reflective Activity 2.3

Before you read on … Think about the definitions and theories outlined above.

Have you heard or read about any of them before? Which?

Do you think any apply to the work you do in your practice?

Do any of the people you see as leaders in your workplace apply any of the theories described above? How?

Do you overtly think about the issue of nursing leadership? If so, why? If not, why not?

If you were to aspire to a leadership role, which of the theories described above might serve you best?

- Creating a space where nurses can get away from the stress of work, at work.

This is done well in the computer development industry but could (and should) be applied in the even more stressful healthcare environments. Rest areas, sleeping or resting pods and quiet or relaxing spaces could be developed. By promoting an environment that actively supports self-care and self-healing, conscious leaders may have a positive impact upon employee satisfaction, reducing sick leave events and costs and limiting absenteeism.

2.5 Summary

This chapter has outlined definitions of leadership and nurse leadership as well as provided a host of information about many leadership theories. The definition of nursing leadership proposed is as follows:

> *Nurse leaders are able to lead, with their values about care and compassion to the fore to inspire, influence and motivate nurse colleagues and other healthcare professionals as they work collaboratively towards the promotion of safe, effective person-centred healthcare and positive, productive collegial relationships.*

For this reason, leadership theories that most closely relate to clinical nursing and nursing-focused leadership are those that support a values-based approach to understanding leadership. These are Authentic/Breakthrough Leadership, Servant Leadership, Shared or Collaborative Leadership, Compassionate Leadership, Conscious Leadership and Congruent Leadership. In addition, the other theoretical approaches presented above will help with a wider concept of leadership. The next chapter will consider what attributes best suit nurse leaders for them to be effective leaders.

> Leaders cannot be turned on and off like an electric fan to blow at the behest of the operator – they behave more like a whirlwind, energised from within, driven by their own values and beliefs.

3

Characteristics of Effective Nurse Leaders

3.1 Introduction

Nurse leaders, in order to be effective, need to display and promote a specific set of skills and attributes. Nursing has had a fraught relationship with leadership, beginning with Florence Nightingale and her abrasive, domineering and controlling approach to leading the female nursing service during and after the Crimean war (Bostridge 2008; Stanley and Sherratt 2010). There she set a poor tone for following nurse leaders to replicate, still she is rightly remembered as a bold, brave, pioneering and revolutionary nurse leader when she had almost no role models to base her pioneering work on. The profession's power struggles for identity and purpose are not new. Abel-Smith's (1960) writing on the historical development of the nursing profession describes the tug for control between employers and nurses, where a desire for professional status and recognition often competes with a managerial discourse. Campaigning for nursing to be recognised as a high-status occupation and profession, Ethel Gordon Manson, matron at St. Bartholomew's Hospital in London combined this with her passion for women's suffrage (Dingwall et al. 1988). Along with Nightingale's example, Manson's influence on the profession's conceptualisation of leadership is often lost today. Yet these are influencers and protagonists from nursing's history, and nursing can build from these examples a vision and concept of nursing leadership for the future. This chapter sets out to identify the attributes that may be considered vital for current effective nurse leaders to be successful.

It also outlines several attributes that are considered counterproductive for nurse leaders to employ.

3.2 Qualities of Effective Nurse Leaders

To be effective and successful, nurse leaders need to be able to influence and engage with others and strive towards operational goals, maintain and live out their values and beliefs, support colleagues and staff and promote safe and effective patient care. To achieve this, nurse leaders need to be emotionally intelligent and well-versed in the hard and soft skills of leadership, recognising that knowledge and clinical skills (hard skills), while vital, are never enough, and that leading people requires excellent people skills (soft skills). Wedderburn Tate (1999) suggested 13 characteristics of effective nurse leaders, divided into 3 subsets:

- **Communication and Language** (proactive language, limited use of jargon and listening).
- **Behaviour** (the Five Fs [friendly, fun, focused, flexible and fast], trust, values, passion, integrity, honesty, to be politically savvy, hold a productive life position and use power well).
- **Development** (which involved homework and networking).

In addition, Stanley et al. (2023) outlined a similar list of attributes of clinical nurse leaders. These were:

- clinical competence/clinical knowledge,
- approachability,
- empowered/motivator or motivated,
- supportive,
- inspires confidence,
- integrity/honesty,
- role model,
- effective communicator,
- visible in practice and
- copes well with change.

Mrayyan et al. (2023) found a number of these attributes in common following their study, with "effective communication," "clinical competence," "approachability," "role modelling" and "support" being dominant in the attributes of clinical nurse leaders in Jordan. In 2022, Jenna Liphart on the web page Nurse Together identified five attributes nurse leaders should have (https://www.nursetogether.com/5-leadership-qualities-every-nurse-should-have/). They were:

- gratitude,
- self-confidence,
- willingness to grow,
- communication skills and
- knowledge.

A number of attributes on the lists above overlap; however, what is more interesting is the wide range of skills identified by each set of authors. Therefore, to fully recognise what sort of attributes nurse leaders need, the section below builds on these attributes dividing them instead into "hard" and "soft" characteristics nurse leaders should display and hold so that they can build effective working relationships in their workplace and lead others effectively.

3.3 Hard Skills for Effective Nurse Leadership

Hard skills describe those that relate to knowledge and the technical aspects of a nurse leader's role.

3.3.1 Advanced Clinical Knowledge and Technical Skills

It goes without saying that if you don't know your job's key functions you will struggle to lead others. As such, successful nurse leaders must be knowledgeable about a range of technical, functional and clinical issues/things including the following.

3.3.2 The Healthcare System, Advocacy and Policy

Vital for knowing your place in the organisation is understanding power, change and the rules that govern your workplace. Knowledge is a form of power and gathering power and influence are central for how leaders function in the world. This implies networking, gaining alliances, control over resources and understanding the system. Great leaders recognise the value of knowledge and the power it conveys, and they use it appropriately. Having wider knowledge about healthcare and policy also equips you with an ability to enter the conversation about decision-making and influencing the direction within the organisation and advocating for patient care.

3.3.3 The Day-to-Day Clinical Activities of Your Role

Leading nurses means being able to effectively undertake the duties and roles of a nurse (Mrayyan et al. 2023). In study after study exploring the leadership attributes of clinical leaders, Stanley (2008, 2019) found that the most common attribute of clinical nurse leaders was that they were seen to have the clinical skills and knowledge to undertake and lead in their role. In research by James (2020), clinical leaders demonstrating values and confidence in clinical activities when mentoring was also considered a key attribute for student nurses. So being seen and viewed by others as leading with a values-based approach, being a congruent leader, has an impact on others (Stanley 2008, 2019; James et al. 2021a; Stanley et al. 2023).

3.3.4 Conflict Management, Networking and Negotiation

You cannot work effectively with others if you cannot negotiate, network or deal well with conflict. Networking is covered in Chapter 7; however, it should be emphasised that using our personal, professional, organisational, strategic and even international networks is central for effective leadership to flourish. Effective nurse leaders establish networks and use them appropriately (Wedderburn Tate 1999; Stanley et al. 2023). They most definitely do not bully, dominate or subvert their colleagues' needs and ideas. Managing conflict swiftly and effectively within teams is essential, and while this may be challenging, it is important for individuals, the collective and patient care. Conflict can quickly spiral to create negative cultures and impact on effective and safe patient care.

3.3.5 Finance, Business and Human Resource Management

These skills and this knowledge are not only of value for managers but can also help clinical-level staff negotiate their way through the world of work, while not vital for all clinical-level nurse leaders, an understanding of these matters can add depth to a leader's skill set.

3.3.6 Strategic Management

Strategy is not something left to generals; seeing the big picture is vital for leaders at all levels. Nurses all too often focus on their ward, their department and their day-to-day activities, without recognising that they are part of a larger system that has wider needs and is influenced and impacted by local, national and international political, financial and economic trends. Having an awareness of this can support influencing and negotiating for improvement and quality issues.

3.3.7 Political Awareness

Acting with integrity requires leaders to be politically savvy. This means leaders need to recognise that the workplace is not an insular microcosm but part of a whole, a place where we have responsibilities to others including patients and as such, we need to build alliances, communicate clearly and support each other to constantly improve patient care. This is made easier if we know the formal and informal pathways and be aware of our influencing powers. Politics can refer to the big "P" politics of the nation or the small "p" politics of the workplace. Both require nurse leaders to be aware of their influence on the workplace and the work environment. This includes speaking up if there are lapses in quality or concerns within the organisation around issue of ethics or quality patient care.

3.3.8 Professional Development

Ongoing education and updating knowledge are central for a leader's development and a requirement of our professional status. Wedderburn Tate (1999, p. 78) called this doing our "*homework,*" suggesting that nurse leaders refresh their knowledge, use reflection and challenge themselves to do better. This can take many forms and is not limited to professional development courses. We learn through engaging in all forms of life, reading, writing, watching TV, being quiet and alone and listening to music. This is important of course in a safety-critical profession and in terms of keeping up with evidence as it emerges. Some would add that developing criticality is also part of this development; reading widely and developing an opinion from the evidence available ensures information is not taken at face value but explored in depth (Henriksen and Børgesen 2016; James et al. 2023). So, by using tacit, implicit and explicit knowledge, leaders can benefit the context and communities they aim to inspire (Henrikson and Børgesen 2016).

3.4 Soft Skills for Effective Leadership

Soft skills relate to the people skills needed to lead. They capture the often delicate and intricate nature of dealing with our colleagues and others. These attributes recognise the importance of having sound people skills. Porter-O'Grady (2017) discusses these skills of effective leadership as a full appreciation of the interconnection of three key areas: people, performance and purpose. Included in these are:

- self-awareness,
- emotional intelligence and social intelligence,
- supporting individuals to perform and feel safe in their work environment,
- valuing each person's strengths and contributions,
- cultivating the potential of individuals and teams and allowing each member of the team to be heard and
- promoting the shared purpose of achieving effective and safe patient care.

These leadership aptitudes focus on nurturing human skills and on supporting nurses to engage with and drive change and innovation (James and Arnold 2022).

3.4.1 Sense of Teamwork and Collaboration

Dealing with teams is addressed in Chapter 6; however, it is clear, given the nature of healthcare work, that being able to work in or lead teams is an especially vital part of a nurse leader's role (Algunmeeyn et al. 2023).

Clearly defined roles and expectations, working towards common goals and being accountable to each other and our responsibilities, as well as coaching and mentoring a culturally diversified workforce are all key attributes of nurse leaders. In addition, a coaching approach can foster a sense of shared vision within the team (James and Arnold 2022). Effective teamwork also implies a supportive team environment with no bullying or deception, and with civil discourse, active listening and collaborative teamworking practices.

3.4.2 Creativity and Innovation

Being mindful and open to new experiences and technologies, nurse leaders can apply innovative and new approaches to leadership. Creativity was not rated highly as a clinical leader attribute in Stanley's (2008, 2019) studies; however, it is clear that being creative in addressing clinical and other issues is an important skill for nurse leaders to hone, in order to grow as leaders. This is especially true in the current constraints and turbulence of today's healthcare systems. Nurse leaders' capacity to address and lead change is very much based on their ability to bring innovations to the fore (Stanley et al. 2023). Indeed, this may be an area where leaders will need to flourish and develop to address the expectations of the future workforce. Christensen et al. (2018) in their literature review identified that the nursing workforce currently consists of:

- "Traditionalists" (born between 1922 and 1945),
- "Baby boomers" (1946–1964),
- "Generation X" (1965–1979),
- "Millennials" (1980–1995) and
- "Generation Z" (born after 1995).

The review highlighted how each generation varies in their expectations and behaviours of nurse leadership. Interestingly they found variations with the nursing profession's newest members "Generation Z," who used digital technology rapidly to answer questions, requiring less direction than previous generations; however, expectations are that the workplace and therefore their leaders be responsive to their needs

(Stanley 2010). Therefore, the teams in which leaders work and engage with are changing, and the leaders are expected to respond with innovative approaches (James et al. 2023).

3.4.3 Dedication to Excellence

What is nursing excellence? There are varying definitions and frameworks globally which aim to define what is meant by excellence within nursing, for example, in the United States, hospitals aiming to achieve Magnet status must evidence and demonstrate a commitment to nursing excellence. This includes sustaining transformational leadership to support nurse engagement, innovation, research and high-quality nursing practice to deliver positive outcomes for staff, patients and the organisation (Valle et al. 2022). In England, the chief nursing officer is supporting a collective leadership approach for excellence in nursing, focusing on transformational leadership, innovation and research. What all agree on is that for nurse leaders, nurturing high standards of evidence-based practice and innovation is important to support staff, patients and the organisation. By applying current and evidence-based practice, demonstrating consistency and passion for the profession and engaging in lifelong learning (a hard skill above), nurse leaders should demonstrate and support an ethos of excellence and forge a sound leadership profile.

3.4.4 Create a Culture That Drives High Reliability and Quality

From the aspects of excellence discussed above, nurse leaders can positively impact patient safety and quality outcomes. From the evidence on patient safety and organisational cultures, we know that leaders can create psychologically safe environments and encourage others to feel comfortable in expressing concerns and ideas to improve quality of care (Aranzamendez et al. 2015; Newman et al. 2017). Of course, both individuals and others in an organisation can influence cultures, but nurse leaders should be aware of this delicate balance and advocate for their professional values to drive positive cultures. This includes a no-blame attitude, asking the difficult questions and creating a fair and transparent culture, where learning from disclosure is encouraged and accountability maintained to support a safe environment (Wilson 2016).

3.4.5 Being Approachable

Wedderburn Tate (1999) described this attribute as the Five Fs: Friendly, Fun, Focused, Flexible and Fast. In research by Stanley (2008, 2019) and later by Mrayyan et al. (2023), clinical leaders were commonly recognised as effective if they were approachable. Implying they treated their colleagues respectfully, were supportive, were honest and communicated well, capturing the core of Wedderburn Tate's Five Fs. Trust is at the heart of being seen as approachable as it is the foundation of a stable relationship. Being cynical, interfering in others' work or being biased all disrupt a stable relationship and lead to leaders being seen as unapproachable. Being approachable means being trustworthy and friendly.

3.4.6 Honesty and Integrity

Effective nurse leaders are honest and have integrity. This was borne out in study after study when nurses were asked to identify the attributes they recognised in clinical nurse leaders (Stanley 2008, 2019; Stanley et al. 2023). Building effective relationships with colleagues and others requires trust and honesty which are vital components of a sound collegial (in fact any) relationship.

3.4.7 Excellent Interpersonal Skills and Effective Emotional Intelligence

This is achieved by using effective written and verbal communication skills, active listening, clarity, confidence and empathy (Mrayyan et al. 2023). Great nurse leaders use jargon sparingly (Wedderburn Tate 1999) and take the initiative using proactive language and deeds. Reactive language and deeds imply a loss of control, while being proactive in our actions and communication suggest responsibility and clear communication. The key here is the application of emotional intelligence (Taylor 2017). Emotional intelligence is outlined in Box 3.1 below. Stanley et al. (2023) also indicate that excellent communication is central to a leader's prospects of success and effectiveness.

Box 3.1   Emotional Intelligence

Goleman (1998b) describes emotional intelligence as the capacity for recognising our own feelings and those of others, for motivating ourselves and for effectively dealing with our own and others' emotions. Salovey and Mayer (1990) describe it as the ability to monitor one's own and others' feelings and emotions, to discriminate among them and to use this information to guide one's thinking and actions. Ellis (2017a) adds that emotional intelligence requires people to be self-aware and understand the reasons behind their emotions and use an emotionally measured and literate response.

Goleman (1998b) reminds us that emotions are a human factor and are also an essential part of who we are, adding that expressing emotions at the right time and in the right place is a concern for most of us. Emotional intelligence means judging when to deal with emotions or when to park them (Brockbank and McGill 2000). Emotional intelligence is about exercising control over these emotions so that our response is tempered by a conscious acknowledgement of the feelings we are experiencing.

The Five Building Blocks of Emotional Intelligence

Self-awareness (of your own feelings)
This is the ability to gauge and understand your emotions and recognise how they will influence your work performance and relationships. It is also about recognising and being realistic regarding your strengths and weaknesses (Ellis 2017a; Mansel and Einion 2019).

Self-management or self-regulation (of your emotions)
This is self-control. It involves the ability to keep disruptive emotions and impulses in check. It requires you to be conscious of your emotions (Ellis 2017b).

Social awareness or empathy (to recognise the feelings of others)
This is about recognising and sensing the emotions of others, understanding their perspective and employing empathy. It is an essential skill for networking and navigating through relationships.

Social skills (to manage emotions in others)
This is a set of skills that build on communication, listening and conflict management. These are skills that build bonds and cooperation.

Motivation
This is the drive to go beyond superficial motivations (money or status) and see the "bigger picture" in building successful and meaningful personal and professional relationships. It captures ideas of optimism and a willingness to be committed to more than just yourself.

3.5 Other Characteristics to Consider

While some of what will be mentioned below is implied above, it is important to clearly state some other characteristics that nurse leaders may display or aspire to in order to be recognised as effective and compassionate nurse leaders. These are as follows.

3.5.1 Courage

Leadership requires courage because brave leaders are never silent when hard choices must be made or when hard paths must be trod. We can't lead if we live in fear of criticism, fear of failure. If we are afraid to go out on a limb, or to the edge, others will fail to recognise the leader within. Theodore Roosevelt said in 1910, "*It is not the critic who counts; not the man who points out how the strong man stumbles, or where the doer of deeds could have done them better. The credit belongs to the man who is actually in the arena, whose face is marred by dust and sweat and blood; who strives valiantly . . . who at the best knows in the end the triumph of high achievement, and who at the worst, if he fails, at least fails while daring greatly.*" This is a mantra supported by Brown (2016), who points out that leadership requires the leader to "show up" or "step up" and dare greatly.

3.5.2 Vulnerability

Leadership requires leaders to be vulnerable because leadership is not about control or command, it is about taking risks and accepting that true courage comes when we are at our most vulnerable. Brown (2016, p. 45) suggests that *"Vulnerability is not winning or losing; it's having the courage to show up and be seen when we have no control over the outcome. . . . vulnerability is not weakness; it's our greatest measure of courage."* Brown (2016, p. 20) adds that, *"Vulnerability is the birthplace of love, belonging, joy, courage, empathy, and creativity. It is the source of hope, empathy, accountability, and authenticity. If we want greater clarity in our purpose . . . vulnerability is the path."* It is therefore the path to effective leadership. There is no courage without vulnerability, and for nurse leaders, uncertainty, risk and emotional exposure test their courage every day. It is scary, but it is the reality of almost every nurse or midwife's work. Leading requires you to be who your values are (the very definition of Congruent Leadership) (Stanley 2019). This takes both vulnerability and courage, risk and failure and all steps on the road to healing, gratitude and joy and to leading greatly.

3.5.3 Compassion and Empathy

Nurse leaders without compassion or empathy cannot remain true to the core values of their role/profession in the health service. To stay the course set by our values means sometimes being vulnerable to naysayers, fools and the ignorant. But pressing on, along a path guided by our core values means risk and ridicule, failure and setbacks. It is from these tests that compassion and empathy grow, and they sit alongside all the other characteristics identified above as vital for nurse leaders to function.

3.6 The Attributes "Least" Likely to Foster Effective Nurse Leadership

As well as identifying the characteristics of effective leaders, it is worth drawing your attention to attributes least likely to be recognised as supporting leadership. They are as follows.

3.6.1 Visionary

Leaders are often recognised for their ability to be visionary to see a future goal and strive for it even in the face of their follower's opposition.

This type of leadership is admirable in some circumstances; however, in a clinical environment having a vision was of less value than holding on to a set of clear values and leading with these to the fore. As such, being visionary is less relevant for nurse leaders (Cook 2001; Stanley, 2008, 2019; Stanley et al. 2023) than other attributes.

3.6.2 Controlling

Being seen as controlling was consistently seen as a turn off when looking for the attributes of effective leaders (Stanley 2008, 2019; Coventry and Russell 2021; Mrayyan et al. 2023; Stanley et al. 2023). While managers may be required to set rules and policies, nurse leaders who had no managerial role were frequently seen to rely on control because they had not mastered other soft (or even hard) skills associated with their leadership role.

3.6.3 Bias/Favouritism

In keeping with a desire to foster honesty and integrity, any behaviour or action that undermined trust and honesty or that looks like deceit, favouritism or biased behaviour was seen to erode the leader's credibility and likeability and the followers' faith in the leader's abilities (Stanley et al. 2023).

3.6.4 Dishonesty

Any leaders who employed a dishonest approach to their leadership role is seen as less valuable as a leader. If a leader was seen as dishonest, their credibility and leadership potential were seriously undermined.

3.7 Summary

This chapter has outlined several attributes and characteristics nurse leaders might display. It suggests that there is a plethora of attributes that have been proposed to identify effective nurse leaders. These include clinical competence/clinical knowledge, approachability, empowerment and being motivated, supportive, inspirational, confident, honest, a role model, an effective communicator, visible in practice, able to cope well with change and show gratitude, self-confident and willing to learn, grow and demonstrate courage and vulnerability. I mean it's a lot. No wonder leadership is hard. Here in this chapter these attributes have been presented as hard and soft skills to help delineate the number of attributes.

Hard skills are described as:

- advanced clinical knowledge and technical skills,
- an understanding of the health system, being an advocate and understanding health policy,
- effectively managing your day-to-day role,
- managing conflict,
- engaging in professional development,
- networking and dealing well with negotiations,
- understanding finance, business and HR issues and
- dealing with strategic management and being politically aware.

Soft skills are described as:

- an ability to deal with teams and collaboration,
- being creative and innovative,
- being dedicated to excellence,
- creating a culture that drives high quality and reliability,
- being approachable,
- being honest and
- applying high-quality emotional intelligence.

In addition, it is proposed that nursing leadership requires the application of emotional intelligence, courage, vulnerability and compassion. A willingness to take risks and embrace failure, heartbreak and hurt and a willingness to take risks and to remain compassionate and show empathy are all central to the core issues that help nurse leaders stand out and be recognised as such. Followers who recognise these core attributes and see the congruence between the leader's actions and values will know they are in the presence of a true nursing leader.

Courage is vital for leaders, and there can be no courage without vulnerability, no understanding without compassion and empathy and no leadership without all four (vulnerability, courage, compassion and empathy).

4

Self-Care for Leadership Effectiveness

4.1 Introduction

This chapter recognises that effective nurse leaders need to find time for themselves in order to lead others. As such it addresses issues of self-care, mindfulness and resilience. Effective leaders as well as leading their team or others, and shouldering their leadership responsibilities, need to take care of themselves. This implies taking time to stop and reflect, practising mindfulness and being able to see their failures as a learning opportunity and their successes and failures together, as a way of building resilience (Ellis 2021).

4.2 Self-Care

Self-care implies self-compassion, and taking care of our own personal/professional needs as a priority. It is the opposite to a slavish devotion to work and sense of self-sacrifice that has dominated nursing's self-perception. Self-care and self-compassion is the ability of individuals, families and communities to promote health, prevent disease, maintain health and cope with illness and disability, with or without the support of a health professional (WHO 2022). Kwon (2023) defines self-care as how nurses promote their own physical and mental health. Eslick et al. (2022) add that self-compassion is directing compassion towards ourselves. Mills et al. (2015) and Sist et al. (2022) agree and suggest that self-care and self-compassion are essential to optimise the care nurses and

Notes On... Nursing Leadership, First Edition. Alison H. James and David Stanley.
© 2024 John Wiley & Sons Ltd. Published 2024 by John Wiley & Sons Ltd.

other health professionals provide to those they care for. Eslick et al. (2022) indicate that self-care builds resilience and enhances a nurse's or health professional's ability to provide compassionate care to others (Kim 2011). Caring for yourself first means you can more effectively care for or lead others. Caring for ourselves is a challenge for nurses as one participant in a study by Andrews et al. (2020) exploring self-care and self-compassion said: "*I always put my patient first, but actually if I've got no self-compassion for myself and I'm not looking after myself I can't give my patients a hundred per cent.*" The Dalai Lama (2000, p. 125) reminds us that:

> For someone to develop genuine compassion towards others, first he or she must have a basis upon which to cultivate compassion, and that basis is the ability to connect to one's own feelings and to care for one's own welfare . . . caring for (or leading) others requires caring for oneself.

A study by Andrews et al. (2020) found that nurses are "*hardwired to be caregivers*" and put others first. The study found that nurses often felt the need to seek permission to be self-compassionate and that many nurses had taken on an identity of self-sacrifice, putting care for others and self-sacrificial behaviours above the notion of self-care and self-compassion. Nurses seem to have been conditioned to diminish their own needs and work slavishly towards the needs of others.

The memoirs and diaries of nurses for centuries are replete with reflections about the obligations they felt and about being compelled to subvert their own needs when caring for others. Nurses have always been willing to put themselves at risk to care for or lead others. Vera Britain's war diary "*Chronicle of youth,*" about her experiences of nursing during the First World War, is replete with examples of the nurse's duty to be ever tired and ever ready to serve. Here is just one example of the depth of self-sacrifice expected of nurses at the time.

> I have just been looking at myself in the glass; tiredness makes one positively ugly. As I have got to be continuously tired for many days to come, I fear at this rate all I ever had of beauty will come to be a thing of the past. Such is war! Even attractiveness must be sacrificed to usefulness (Bishop and Smart 1982, p. 272).

Self-sacrifice remains a powerful theme in modern nursing; this was evident in the way nurses and other health professionals were portrayed during the COVID-19 outbreak. Nurses were called upon to work long hours and many gave their lives (as did other health professionals) while caring for others. The symbol of angel wings became a dominant feature on social media with imagery suggestive of nurses again being self-sacrificial heroines, angels, that stood as a motivational force for nursing recruitment and practice and as a symbol the community at large took to represent self-sacrifice in the face of the pandemic. However, failing to provide self-care in the healthcare service has consequences for health professionals, patients, the organisation and the health service in general. Nurse leaders need to recognise that without reasonable self-care, their longevity or effectiveness as leaders will be limited. The consequences of a lack of self-care for nurses and nurse leaders are listed below:

- Fewer healthier, happier staff at work.
- Less willing or able followers.
- Tired leaders who make poor decisions.
- Shorter leadership careers.
- Leaders with more work-induced health issues (burnout/illness/stress).
- Leaders who feel less engaged with their workplace, colleagues or other healthcare staff and client/patients.
- Resentment and disillusionment with work.
- Greater numbers of staff who become burnt out, depressed, disengaged or disillusioned with their careers.
- More staff and leader resignations due to burnout, depression or stress-related injuries.

4.3 Caring for Self

In a study by Melnyk et al. (2018), over half of their study respondents reported less than optimal physical or mental health with a correlation between poor health and workplace errors, pointing towards a lack of self-care as the cause. To counter our history and to work towards a better future, we need to understand the concept of self-care. Healthcare is provided in a host of clinical environments, most of which feature change and stress as constant elements, and these can have negative impacts on the nurse leader's well-being and health (both physical and mental) and may result in feelings of low self-worth or resentment. In a recent study of over 300 nurses by Ross et al. (2019), almost half of their study participants reported the negative effects of work stress impacting their eating habits and as a result more than half were overweight or obese. In addition, Davidson et al. (2018) noted that nurses have a higher suicide rate than the national average in the United States. In Korea, the practice of nurse "hazing" has been identified as having a detrimental impact on nurses and their self-worth, with the national suicide rate amongst nurses growing along with the advent of a *taeum* (burn-to-ashes) culture. This sees senior nurses getting special privileges and hierarchical advantages and a parallel growth in the harassment and bullying of junior nurses with 65% of nurses indicating they have experienced bullying in Korea (Jeong 2018; Kim and Sim 2021). Bullying remains an issue in all areas of nursing across the globe with a plethora of publications attesting to the score of colleague-on-colleague trauma or horizontal violence being practiced (Mikaelian and Stanley 2016; Budden et al. 2017; MacDonald et al. 2022). Understanding self-care and self-compassion may help alleviate and diminish the incidence of bullying or at least enable nurse leaders to focus on their own needs and employ ways to care for themselves as energetically as they are required to care for others and lead their teams.

Self-care can be described as how nurse leaders promote their own physical and mental health needs. Eslick et al. (2022) add that self-compassion occurs when nurses direct compassion towards themselves and that self-compassion builds resilience. Lamothe et al. (2014) are of the view that in addition to resilience, self-compassion can decrease stress, improve staff well-being and have a positive impact on the quality of patient care. The WHO (2022) and Sist et al. (2022) suggest that it is essential that nurses take steps to engage in activities to establish and maintain their own health. Sist et al. (2022) adds that self-care is vital so that nurses can optimise the care they provide and prevent serious errors in care or adverse consequences for their own health. The main element of self-care focuses on the relationship the nurse and nurse leader have with themselves. Establishing a self-focused relationship requires self-knowledge, insights into our individual personality type, an understanding of how we cope with change and stress and an understanding of our own personal resources when faced with new and demanding or challenging situations.

4.4 Building Self-Care and Self-Compassion

In order to protect nurses from burnout and workplace stress, self-care and self-compassion need to be promoted. Vidal-Blanco et al. (2018) found in a study exploring the quality of work life and self-care within nursing that organisational factors were significant barriers to implementing effective self-care. In addition, Couser, Chesak and Cutshall (2020) recognised that a course to promote self-care was needed to reduce the impact of burnout negatively impacting on staff health and the quality of patient care. In Holland, the Excellent Care Program (de Kok et al. 2023) supports the notion and practice of facilitating enhanced leadership education and training to address the importance of a positive work environment. There is a plethora of approaches that may be used to promote self-care and self-compassion, and there seems to be a proliferation of in-service or short courses seeking to retrofit health professionals with strategies for coping with stress and developing greater self-care habits. All are aimed at providing manageable and useful self-care tools to prevent stress and improve workforce retention, with the quality and direction of leadership a key element in all of them.

To achieve self-care, nurse leaders should aim to get sufficient exercise to maintain their fitness and eat a suitable, healthy varied diet, high in fibre and with enough energy to facilitate the mental and physical work required in a nurse leader's working day. Sleep although often ignored and difficult to secure in many nurse leaders' employment situations is equally vital, with the need to get adequate rest and sleep often overlooked as a tool to maintain effective self-care. Enough sleep and a suitable diet and exercise should all be considered vital for any health professional to deal with their work and personal life.

In addition, self-care requires time for personal reflection (Berman et al. 2021) with adequate "down time" allowing health professionals to recharge their batteries and spend quality time with their families and loved ones. Wedderburn Tate (1999) puts this simply suggesting that nurses and nurse leaders need to take lots of holidays. Health professionals should avoid unhealthy patterns of behaviour such as negative self-talk, or negative thinking, wasting time on negative body image ideation or self-image shaming, and poor social behaviours that have detrimental effects on our bodies' physical state (e.g. smoking, excessive drinking of alcohol and drug abuse).

4.5 Mindfulness

Sitzman and Watson (2018) suggest that incorporating mindfulness into the practice of nursing care is directly linked to the cultivation of a deep and lasting understanding between the nurse and patient and this applies to the activity of nurse leadership and understanding between the leader and the led. Crane and Ward (2016) suggest that the key to self-care is self-awareness, and they recommend undertaking a self-inventory of our feelings and coping strategies in anticipation of having to face a challenging situation or following a stressful event. Wedderburn Tate (1999) again makes this point simply by suggesting that nurse leaders need to have active "crap" detectors. The aim is to gain greater insight into how leaders/nurses respond to challenges and plan strategies to manage our feelings and respond more effectively to them. Mindfulness is closely related to meditation, which is also a key attribute of becoming self-aware (Crane and Ward 2016). Mindful strategies include:

- Mindful self-compassion (MSC) is an eight-week training program in mindfulness and meditation technique with a focus on loving/kindness and meditation aimed to enhance self-compassion (Delaney 2018).
- Mindful self-care and resilience (MSCR) is a four-week training intervention in mindfulness meditation techniques that includes educational workshops on compassion fatigue and resilience (Craigie et al. 2016; Slatyer et al. 2018).
- Mindfulness-based stress reduction (MBSR) involves mindfulness and self-compassion training (Foureur et al. 2013; Mahon et al. 2017).
- Mindful prostration is a popular practice among Korean Buddhists and involved 108 prostrations. Its focus is on humility and sincerity with the practice seen as a conversation between the body and the mind (Kim 2018).
- Sutra copying is based in a Buddhist sutra that focuses on reading with the eyes, memorising by mouth, writing by hand and bearing in mind.

The process takes time, concentration and devotion, with practitioners claiming the process brings calmness and comfort (Kim 2017).

- Cultivating an attitude of gratitude is a popular idea for counteracting some of the stresses and challenges of life. A way to do this is to write a gratitude journal, where items that result in gratitude are written down each day. The idea is that this process will lead to feelings of appreciation and gratitude. Crane and Ward (2016) recommend building expressions of gratitude into general discussions and even staff meetings.

4.6 Resilience

Resilience is about your capacity to bounce back from knocks, from doubt and from setbacks. The world will not always fall at your feet. It will often be beset with difficulties, challenges and noxious others, who may throw thorns in your path. Resilience describes your capacity to be elastic, to be tough and to withstand or spring back from difficulties. Nurses are expected to be resilient, and the term has become increasingly present, especially since the COVID-19 pandemic in narratives and research in the nursing press. However, there is also criticism of the sometimes over-reliance on individual resilience to compensate for lack of organisational resources and support, such as adequate staffing and conditions (Traynor 2017). Therefore, nurse leaders must not place too high expectations, that we can face high levels of stress and unacceptable conditions in our work environment. It is important that nurse leaders identify when staff may be exhausted and under strain. When personal resilience is not supported by organisational responsibility, nurse leaders can be the negotiating force to advocate for balanced conditions.

Wedderburn Tate (1999) describes resilient leaders as being coated in rubber, but even rubber can deteriorate and fail or be run through with thorns. Perhaps resilience is more like one of those inflatable bumper balls that people wear to play soccer or to roll down hills safely. You can put them on when needed, inflate or deflate them and use them to keep you safe when the outside world gets bumpy or when you need more bounce. The Bounce Back Project (2023) (https://www.feelinggoodmn.org/what-we-do/bounce-back-project-/5-pillars-of-resilience/#:~:text=Resilience%20is%20made%20up%20of,Care%2C%20Positive%20Relationships%20and%20Purpose) suggests that resilience is made up of five pillars: **Self Awareness, Mindfulness, Self-Care, Positive Relationships** and **Purpose** and that by strengthening these pillars, we can become more resilient. Instead of experiencing an overwhelming downward spiral when we encounter stress in our lives, these five pillars work together to lift us up out of the chaos we are feeling. The Bounce Back Project (2023) adds that by applying a few simple tools we can build our sense of self and thicken our resilient armour or inflate our bumper ball. These include showing gratitude, random acts of kindness, staying connected with our family, friends, and others, staying mindful and remaining focused on a purpose.

Reflective Activity 4.1

Before you read on … Reflect upon the attributes outlined above.
  Are there any you disagree with?
  Are they any you would add to the list?
  Discuss the attributes you see as central to a nurse leader's role with a colleague or you ward/clinical leader. Do they agree with you?
  What attributes do they see as vital for a nurse leader to be effective?

4.7 Summary

If nurse leaders are to capture even a part of the attributes required to lead as outlined in Chapter 3, they will need to have a firm grasp of their own self-care or self-compassion needs. Nurse leaders should apply mindfulness and their own personal resilience to build a strong sense of self and insight into their own values.

5

Leadership for Innovation and Change

5.1 Introduction

Change seems to be an almost unrelenting feature of the health service industry (Essen and Lindblad 2013) and as West et al. (2017, p. 1) indicate, "only innovation can enable modern health care organisations and systems to meet the radically changing needs and expectations of the communities they serve." However, this needs to be balanced because during our time working in the National Health Service (in the United Kingdom), and to a lesser extent in other health services, modifications to the structure of the service felt like almost biannual events. Healthcare organisations and hospital divisions were amalgamated or disbanded, rebranded or dissolved with little real impact on the frontline service offered by clinically based staff, apart from never-ending disruptions and feelings of disempowerment. The after-effects of the COVID-19 pandemic seem only to have exacerbated the process and advent of change.

The issue is that organisations, particularly those such as hospitals or those that deal with healthcare concerns, are not like factories. They are communities of people and therefore they behave just like other communities. People are the core resource of the health service and even with the advent and entrenchment of technology, people are still, and will always be, central to the health industry and the leadership of these people is pivotal to how the organisations will function. Nurses, although the largest healthcare group in most countries, have commonly failed to understand how change can be managed and may still fail to recognise

Notes On... Nursing Leadership, First Edition. Alison H. James and David Stanley.
© 2024 John Wiley & Sons Ltd. Published 2024 by John Wiley & Sons Ltd.

that they can direct or influence change, rather than be passive respondents to the forces about them.

In nursing and healthcare, as in the wider community, there are a number of potential reactions to change, and it is these very differences that provide the fuel to drive the life of the organisation or community. It is these very differences that are essential if a community is going to continue to adapt to the world about it, to change, or in other words to develop and react to new situations. Change is a necessary condition of survival whether for individuals, communities or organisations. Differences are a necessary ingredient for change and stimulate a never-ending search for improvement. Improving quality in healthcare involves changing the way things are done, changing processes and the behaviour of people and teams of people. The challenge for any one of us is to harness the energy and thrust of differences so that the individual, community or organisation does not disintegrate during the process of change but develops and grows.

Without change we will wither and die, so from this perspective change needs to be embraced and managed. By that we mean evaluating the effects of change, sustaining the change if it is effective and positive and recognising when change needs to meet resistance or redirection. There are ways we can help change come about without destruction, dispute, hostility and division. This chapter suggests a range of tools that can be used to successfully manage change. Babine et al. (2016, p. 40) support this view, indicating that it is a key part of the clinical nurse leader's role to engage in "systems management" that supports the implementation of sustainable practice change.

This chapter will focus on leading change and innovation in practice. It will enable nurse leaders to recognise the steps for identifying areas where change is needed, to plan, implement and evaluate the change. An overview of some models of change will be introduced, and the challenges and potential barriers, such as organisational cultures and the importance of developing networks of support and approaches to networking, are presented. It will draw on examples from clinical practice that demonstrate how leadership has positively impacted upon the quality of patient care and why it is important for the future of the nursing profession.

> Innovation and change are the domains of leaders in the modern health service; managers are important and leaders are vital.

5.2 Tools for Change

A number of tools can be used to support change. Each will be explored in this section. However, before these are outlined it should be noted that even with effective tools, it does not mean that change, at least planned change, will result. The models will help, but in the end, it may depend on the circumstances and attitude with which they are used, as much as your skill with the tools and leading the change. Iles (2011a) makes it clear that to be beneficial, change needs to be approached with care, courage and enthusiasm. Therefore, tools are merely methods of supporting your approach to change, not the magic remedy for success. Iles (2011a, p. 22) sees "conversation" as central to this process and reminds change agents (leaders) that simple, empathetic, engaging conversations that bring people into the process of change are vital for the outcome to be positive. This process requires listening as much as talking.

5.2.1 SWOT Analysis

A SWOT analysis can be used as a personal reflection tool or as an organisational management and change management tool. By looking at an organisation's strengths, weaknesses, opportunities and threats, you may be able to analyse the current direction of the organisation (ward/clinical area/workplace), formulate future goals and objectives, or analyse specific situations, ideas, groups or activities. Then, once the assessment is made, ask yourself, can you change or challenge the threats or consider how threats can be changed to opportunities or weaknesses to strengths?

The process requires scrupulous honesty and the capacity to be open and look at the threats (Mind Tools 2023; https://www.mindtools.com/amtbj63/swot-analysis). By looking at these you may be able to foresee the obstacles to change. The four parts to a SWOT analysis are:

- Strengths: What are the strengths of your organisation (ward/unit)? In what areas does it function well?
- Weaknesses: What are the weak points in your organisation (ward/unit/department)?
- Opportunities: Are there circumstances present that create openings and the potential for positive change?
- Threats: Are there other circumstances that could threaten or jeopardise your organisation?

5.2.2 Stakeholder Analysis

Stakeholder analysis is used to develop a profile of the people vital for the change to be achieved. These are the people central or peripheral to the proposed change. When using the model, ensure you avoid using real names (to avoid identifying actual individuals and causing potential offence) but do consider the characteristics of the individuals that you see as stakeholders, to assess their capacity to be helpful, ambivalent or obstructive. Think carefully about why you see people having certain attributes. In the model, people are likened to three animal types: sheep, donkeys or lions. Sheep will follow; donkeys will resist, be sceptical and even work against change; and lions will adopt to or champion the change. This analysis allows you to consider who has low tolerance to change. Who are likely to be the adventurous types, who look for a challenge, who the sceptics may be and who the adaptors and saboteurs are. Working these out will profit from the proposed change greatly as it may allow leaders to target known agitators or develop a more collaborative or inclusive strategy for change to diminish resistance and share ownership (Varvasovszky and Brugha 2000).

5.2.3 Pettigrew's Change Model

The core of Andrew Pettigrew's model emphasises the importance of a broad, contextual approach to change. Pettigrew felt that an analysis of change should not just look at the processes of change but also at the political features of an organisation, and the history and cultural context in which the change might take place (Pettigrew and Whipp 1998). The model offers a continuous interplay between the ideas about the context of change, the process of change and the content of change (Pettigrew et al. 2001).

The usefulness of this model is that it reminds the leader to consider the complexities of an organisation, and that it is commonly influenced by characteristics in the internal and external environment. Pettigrew defined the context as the "why and when" of change, differentiating between the inner and outer aspects of the context (outer might be the prevailing economic circumstances and the social and political climate at the time. Inner might refer to the resources, structure, culture and local politics). Content is described as the "what" of change and is concerned with areas of transformation, that is "what" is to be changed. The process is described as the "how" of change and refers to how the change will be made to come about, what actions are needed, who will do what and how things will get done.

5.2.4   The Change Management Iceberg

Wilfried Kruger developed the change management iceberg as a process to deal with change and the barriers to change. Kruger's view (Ackerman-Anderson and Anderson 2001) is that many leaders consider the tip of the iceberg (cost, quality and time) as significant issues. However, the proposed change is also influenced by other issues – below the surface. These are the management of perceptions and beliefs about the proposed change and issues of power and politics.

These issues imply that more needs to be understood about the proposed change for it to be implemented successfully. Dealing with the types of barriers that arise and how the change can be implemented is dependent on the kind or type of change and the strategy of change that is followed or applied. The kind of change may focus on information systems/processes/policies etc. which can be difficult to implement, but only scratch the surface in terms of their impact on the iceberg. They can also focus on wider issues such as values/mindsets/capabilities, which can result in more profound change and be even more difficult to initiate or suffer from more ingrained barriers. The iceberg model also offers insight into the types of people who might be involved in the change, and like the stakeholder analysis, Kruger involves people in the change assessment.

The change management iceberg model recognises that change is a constant feature of a manager's (leader's) task, but that superficial (tip of the iceberg) issue management can only achieve results on a limited level (structural change). For greater impact and control of the change, wider issues such as the interpersonal and behavioural dimensions, cultural dimensions, power and politics, perceptions and beliefs need to be considered. The model supports the concept of a complete and thorough assessment of the barriers that may impact the change, so the change is likely to be implemented with a greater chance of success.

5.2.5   PEST or STEP

The PEST (political, economic, social and technological) analysis (sometimes called STEP by changing the letters or words about) is useful as an overall environmental scan for an organisation and while included here is not generally as useful as some of the other change tools at a local or ward-based level. It is very useful to gain an overview of the "health," sustainability or resilience of an organisation.

The factors assessed are:

1) Political: tax policy, employment laws, environmental regulations, trade restrictions and tariffs, political stability.
2) Economic: economic growth, interest rates, exchange rates, inflation rate.
3) Social: health consciousness, population growth rate, age distribution, career attitudes, emphasis on safety and generational make-up of the workforce.
4) Technological: R&D activity, automation, technological incentives, rate of technological change.

A PEST analysis may take some time and be undertaken by a range of individuals with specialist skills in the various areas suggested. It may also be used in conjunction with a range of other change management tools, for example, SWOT analysis (Mind Tools 2023; https://www.mindtools.com/aqa3q37/pest-analysis).

5.2.6   Kotter's Eight-Stage Change Process

Kotter's (1996) model is quite simple: it offers an eight-stage process for progressing change, offering a pattern or map that can support and direct clinical leaders and others when initiating or planning change (Jones and Bennett 2018). The steps are:

1) Establish a sense of urgency.
2) Create a guiding coalition (involve people at all levels to establish a shared vision and address specific needs).
3) Develop a vision and strategy (this needs to work towards the planned change).
4) Communicate the change/vision to others.
5) Empower employees for action (let people know that their opinions matter).

6) Strive for short-term wins (good leadership is essential for short-term achievements).
7) Consolidate gains and produce more change (address resistance and strengthen leadership approaches).
8) Anchor new approaches in the culture.

5.2.7 Nominal Group Technique

Nominal group technique is an excellent change tool for helping groups to solve problems or propose changes for themselves. It may not be as useful for driving change through, but it is very handy for identifying where scarce resources and personnel with limited time can focus their energies. It is also an excellent tool for helping to engage wide numbers of people in the change process. The tool is useful for establishing what problems exist and what priority is placed on various competing issues. Significantly, it employs the stakeholders who take part in the process of decision-making so that the priority problems or change issues have been identified from within the stakeholder group. The process for nominal group technique is relatively simple, but it takes time to set up and requires the majority of the stakeholders to engage in it for it to be successful. Have all the stakeholders gather or meet in some way, then follow the steps below:

- Ask the group to split into small groups and discuss the first question: "What are the problems with . . ." or "what are the bad things with . . ." (you can add the relevant problem/issue here). Use butchers' paper to record the discussion. Establish a clear time frame. Once the groups are finished, ask them to post up their lists for all the other groups to read. Make sure the group's discussion sticks to the core questions.
- Ask the same small groups to discuss the second question: "What are the good things about . . ." Again, give the small groups some butchers' paper to record their lists and a suitable time frame, and once they are finished, again post the "good things" list on a wall for all the groups to read. This process can take some time.
- Ask the whole group to review the small group "problems" and "good" points listed.
- Ask them to read and discuss them informally as they review what the other groups have written. Ask everyone to vote for their top three problems.

- To do this, offer a large number of felt-tip pens and have each person vote for the three main problems by ranking them "3," "2" and "1." After everyone has "voted," calculate the results, with the highest number being the issue of most concern to the majority of participants (stakeholders).

In this way the whole group has considered all the issues and decided themselves what the primary three issues are. This can be very empowering for stakeholders. The process isn't over though; the final step is to ask stakeholders to focus only on these three problems. In their small groups again, ask them to propose potential solutions.

This process will identify where the good (this is important to retain a fair perspective on the issues being discussed) and bad things about an issue/problem are and what might be done about them. The problem will still need to be addressed, but using this approach means that implementing change (that is often suggested by the stakeholders) has a greater chance of success as they have had a significant hand in identifying the issues and the potential solution. In addition, they have had a public and detailed opportunity to express their feelings and issues with people often in a position to support or direct resources for change (Sample 1984).

5.2.8 Process Re-Engineering

Process re-engineering is all about sticky notes! (They are small, usually yellow, low-adhesive notes that can be removed and repositioned easily.) The process involves deciding on an issue or process that you would like to change. Gather together all the key stakeholders in one place. Give out a stack of different coloured sticky notes for each participant. Depending on the process under review and number of participants, it may be wise to break the large group into smaller groups. But usually, the group needs to have representation from all areas involved in the process under review for it to be successfully assessed.

The first step is to brainstorm what the issues/problems/current processes are. These are then written on separate sticky notes, breaking everything down into its component parts. Then with everyone's input, put the issue/problem/process back together using the sticky notes to manipulate the process, make changes or suggest new ways to deliver the desired outcome. Discussion is vital, as is physically moving the sticky notes about to see if/how a new process evolves. It may require a great deal of creativity and may also need people to suspend established ideas about how processes are traditionally done. The process has the potential to offer a whole new solution to significant problems or issues. It may point to restructuring and can be used in conjunction with other change management tools. This process can also be an empowering tool and often brings all the stakeholders together by valuing everyone's input, like a team building exercise. As such, a key to the process is skilful facilitation of the sticky note activity.

5.2.9   Force Field Analysis (FFA)

Force Field Analysis (FFA) has a clear advantage over the other models in relation to its use in the health arena; that is, it allows the leader to place themselves clearly in the picture and see their part in the process of change. The other advantage of FFA is that it is very easy to follow and use. Brager and Holloway (1992) described it as a tool for assessing the prospects of organisational change and Egan (1990) summed this up by describing FFA as an analysis of the major obstacles to, and resources for, the implementation of strategies and plans for change. It was developed because it was clear that stability within a social system is dynamic, rather than static, and the result of opposing and constraining forces. Lewin (1951) speculated that these operated to produce what we see or sense as stability. Changes occur when the forces shift, thus causing a disruption in the system's equilibrium. Lewin's model is therefore a way of listing, discussing and dealing with the forces that make possible or obstruct change (Jones and Bennett 2018). An analysis of these forces helps generate options that can help achieve or work against the objectives:

- Restraining forces: that work against the change.
- Driving forces or facilitating forces: that work for or facilitate change.

Analysing these forces can determine if a solution can get the support needed, identify obstacles to successful solutions, suggest actions to reduce the strength of the obstacles and determine where the leader's part in the change process might be and will be useful for an individual or for an organisation. The way to identify either restraining or driving forces is to employ other change tools (such as a SWOT analysis) or to use mind maps, brainstorming, consider the advantages and disadvantages of the change, explore key issues, or to follow "check or think" steps where you stop, question and consider what you have done, and re-plan as required.

Also consider social support and challenges and seek advice from others (e.g. experts, people who may have more experience or insights than you). Seek feedback on performance or get confirmation that you are on the right track, undertake education and training as this may provide you with the information you are looking for or give you more information to place you in a stronger position and undertake research and development to discover if someone else has faced this issue before. In effect, an FFA is a judged look at the potential future, saving some grief as you become forewarned.

5.2.10   Initiating, Envisioning, Playing, Sustaining: A Theoretical Synthesis for Change

This model offers a cyclical approach to change with four stages.

1) The first is for the change to be "initiated": setting goals and/or stating the problem.
2) The second stage is "envisioning": where a vision for the future is outlined.
3) The third stage is "playing": the vision and goals are tested throughout the organisation. The implication is that the "leader" observes how the vision and goals are being implemented and makes appropriate adjustments to lead the followers to success.
4) The final stage is "sustaining": this implies that the change has taken root and with evaluation can be seen to be sustained change.

It is concluded that the process never really stops as evaluation and initiation are ongoing, so that as new problems arise and new goals are set, the stages renew and develop (Edgehouse et al. 2007).

Reflective Activity 5.1

Before you read on ... The change management models offered above may also be applied to other aspects of your life.

Choose SWOT analysis and apply it to a professional or personal issue you may be facing now.

What are the advantages and disadvantages of the SWOT analysis? Would other models be more or less useful for the issues you have considered?

5.2.11 Seven S-Action Words Model for Organisational Change

The seven S-action words are words leaders can use to develop strategies to develop and lead change. These are scan, select, sense, sicken, sift, speak and spread. As such, leaders need to understand that to move from the status quo to successful change they need to use and employ the various S-action words in their change model (Edgehouse et al. 2007).

5.2.12 Beckhard and Harris's Change Equation

This model, in keeping with sound mathematical principles, uses a set of variables to assess resistance to change. The model places staff engagement at its heart with an equation offering a solution to resistance (R) with dissatisfaction (D) and the present situation, a vision (V) for what can be achieved, and the first steps (F) taken towards the vision (Jones and Bennett 2018). All leading to a path to overcome resistance (R). The model is expressed as:

$$D \times V \times F > R$$

5.2.13 People-Mover Change Model: Effectively Transforming an Organisation

This model has four parts: reflective motivation, team-based preparation, strategy implementation and evaluation.

1) The model begins with the leader asking themselves vital or key questions about the planned change. The aim is to identify passion for the proposed change.
2) The next step is to select partners (team members) who will work with the leader to support the change.
3) In the third stage, strategy implementation, the change is communicated to others.
4) Finally, the impact of the change is evaluated. The process is about moving people along by motivating them and winning them over to the proposed change (Edgehouse et al. 2007).

5.2.14 Instituting Organisational Change: A Examination of Environmental Influences

In this model, it is suggested that sustainable change is best achieved if the environment is most suitable for change to occur. It is proposed that organisations need to have:

1) a high value placed on change,
2) a safe environment for change to occur and
3) open dialogue with those affected by change.

It implies that a change-willing organisation will be prepared to assess its strengths, weaknesses and resources, plan for future development and then apply itself to effective change (Edgehouse et al. 2007).

5.3 Change Is Never Simple Even with a Model

There are many change management models, and many approaches overlap or encroach on the methods and theories of others. In this regard, choosing a model or set of change models is crucial if clinical leaders are to make effective plans for change. However, change is not an easy thing to effect, and it is never just a matter of selecting or applying a change model (Stanley, Bennett and James 2023). Clark (2008) suggests that change fails because either strategy, operations or people are to blame. Mostly, he claims it is people who negatively affect change. However, successful change requires all three areas to function effectively, so choosing an appropriate change model is only part of the issue.

Banutu-Gomez and Banutu-Gomez (2007) also suggest that several factors are important for leaders to bring about organisational change. These are:

1) having a vision of where you want to go,
2) having a clear sense of their goals,
3) valuing others' skills and experiences,
4) courageously accepting responsibility for problems,
5) clearly communicating,
6) challenging the status quo,
7) empowering others,
8) setting examples and showing the way,
9) motivating others and
10) positively influencing the culture of an organisation.

As mentioned, understanding the change management models may not be enough and as Banutu-Gomez and Banutu-Gomez (2007) suggest, this is not even mentioned in their important factors for bringing about organisational change. However, it is argued here that having some change management literacy is vital, because understanding the steps of a change model allows novice leaders a framework for planning and assessing their part in change and the steps and actions needed to be successful. Health professionals are not routinely taught change models, and yet change is a central part of the health service environment. Therefore, if nurse leaders are to influence and support better quality care, they need to know and be literate with models for change, as well as having an insight into some of the other key factors outlined (Banutu-Gomez and Banutu-Gomez 2007).

5.4 Resistance to Change

In the health arena, change is often difficult to implement because of the complexity of our systems and frequently faces strong resistance due to often more human factors. This may be the result of a culture where hierarchical structures and constant rounds of change produce scepticism on unprecedented levels. Cultures of resistance can have negative consequences, and this has been evidenced in instances of failure in care such as the Mid Staffordshire report by Francis (2013).

Therefore, if leaders are to facilitate change, they need to be aware that resistance is common, and they should be aware of both its likely cause and also strategies for how resistance can be combated or acknowledged. Knowing the cultures of the organisation and team is therefore a key insight for the nurse leader, and the groundwork is needed before any thoughts of implementing change can begin. Methods to support staff accept or be involved in change may include coaching, education and updating knowledge, or action learning, and these support a change in attitudes and motivation for change (James and Arnold 2022).

The paradox for leaders is to manage the change by having a degree of control on the process while also allowing individuals to be innovative. There are many reasons why individuals are resistant to change, and this may be due to fear of the personal impact of change.

Some people resist change because they display:

- Self-interest and conflicting agendas: For other health professionals change is resisted because it is not seen to be in their best interests to support it (Jones and Bennett 2018). There may be fear of a loss of power, influence, status, money or position, and Daft (2000), Weihrich and Koontz (1993) and Griffin (1993) suggest that fear of loss may be the greatest obstacle to change within organisations. Change requires a readjustment and this, good or bad, implies an increase in stress (Dent and Galloway-Goldberg 1999).
- Uncertainty: Announcing a change and then expecting people to follow organisations on journeys into the unknown, without providing information or insight, remains a main reason for people to offer resistance to planned change. Fear and uncertainty are again the net result (Griffin 1993; Weihrich and Koontz 1993; Daft 2000).
- Diverging points of view: Festinger (1957) labelled this issue "cognitive dissonance." The issue is that what the managers see as an appropriate change may not be seen as a change that is considered appropriate by employees or staff leading to potential conflict.
- Ownership: (or lack of ownership) may help some participants in the change to feel disconnected. Understanding the purpose of the change is a key factor in bringing participants along. Bringing in change "because you can," because you have authority over others, may fail.
- Recognising the drivers: People may resist change simply because they see the change as a threat to their self-worth or personal integrity.

People like being in control or consulted; they do not feel comfortable if their values and beliefs are under threat or at risk of assault.

- Some people just don't like change: It needs to be acknowledged that some people with specific personality types are more inclined to be resistant to change than others. Individuals bring with them their own beliefs, values, support systems, cognitive levels, personality types, languages, behaviours, cultural influences, maturity levels, emotional intelligence levels, emotions and emotional needs, and in the end some people have a low tolerance for change (Jones and Bennett 2018).
- Recognising denial, reflecting time: When faced with change people commonly go into an initial period of denial (Rashford and Coghlan 1994). This is normal, as adjusting to the concept and reality of change takes time, and denial offers a period of reflection and thought. It is during this time that information should be provided, explanations offered and time given for the proposal(s) to take form in people's minds.

5.5   Successfully Dealing with Change

Marquis and Hudson (2021) and Curtis and White (2002) suggest that leaders should not only expect resistance but also be prepared to deal with it when it occurs. They also suggest the following points for change to be successfully introduced:

- Introduce change slowly.
- Facilitate the participation of all involved.
- Facilitate ownership, on a cognitive level, by participants in the proposed change.
- Ensure participants are invested in the process of change.
- Provide information about the proposed change early to allow people to adjust and accept or take part in the changes.
- Facilitate open and honest communication. This will allow for trust and limit misunderstandings.
- Offer support (psychological/emotional/informational) for people struggling with the proposed changes.
- Dignam et al. (2012) and Stanley and Stanley (2018) suggest that collaboration is essential for change to be successful, employing an

external change agent as an objective outsider may be able to facilitate the change more dispassionately. Although the risk here is that they may also be seen with cynicism or mistrust if they do not follow the points above.

Reflective Activity 5.2

Before you read on... Think about why some people may be resistant to change. Do you think nurses and other health professionals are generally risk-takers or generally conservative by nature?
What has been your personal attitude to changes you have been involved with?
Speak with some colleagues about changes that have occurred in the past.
How did your colleagues cope?
How were these changes viewed then, and what impact do they have now?

Recognising that resistance may be prevalent and acknowledging the complexities of planning and implementing a program of change, Robbins et al. (2001) suggest that to successfully bring about change, there needs to be a clearly defined action plan, adequate resources to facilitate the planned change, the incentive to change, the skills to push through what is required and a vision that is shared with all stakeholders of what is to be achieved. If confusion, anxiety and frustration are to be avoided and if resistance is to be addressed or minimised, planning the change process requires the application of a suitable change model and the steps Robbins et al. (2001) suggest.

5.6 Leadership, Innovation and Change are Linked

Innovation, addressing change and goal setting or vision are all linked to a number of perspectives of leadership. However, the degree to which this is true is very much dependent on the theoretical principles that underpin the leader's approach to leadership and the organisation's hope and investment in the leader's outcome. Transformational leadership theory is very much based on the leader's vision and outcomes of leadership that realise change. Indeed, this theoretical approach was at the core of the change agenda in the NHS during the 1990s and early 2000s. This does not mean that the change or innovations proposed were driven by a focus on organisational values; in fact the main drivers were economic and management focused platforms. It is proposed here that the generation of leadership that brings about change and improvements in care are most relevant when supported by a values-based approach to leadership more commonly seen with nurse leaders. West et al. (2017) propose that if leaders bring the core elements of compassion to their leadership style (attending, understanding, empathising and helping) as such, healthcare leaders can have a positive impact on the quality of care, patient safety, the patient's experience, resource efficiency and the well-being of staff and foster greater innovation. Indeed, West et al. (2017), Stanley (2008, 2019) and Stanley, Bennett and James (2023) are all of the view that a values-based leadership approach has far greater opportunity to lead values-based change, and nurse leaders are very much at the forefront of finding, developing and enacting innovations in practice or the clinical domain to improve the working life of their colleagues and/or clients/patients.

It is proposed that the most relevant changes and innovations in practice have only come about because nurses involved in frontline care practice have seen and suggested the changes that make a real difference to the client/patient's wellbeing. Changes and developments in wound care, skin care, hydration, elimination and comfort with the advent of better-quality beds have all come from nurses in frontline roles who have seen care deficits and who have forged a way to make care better.

This is because values-based nurse leadership approaches promote leaders who nurture a culture of care and compassion and support a culture where values embody the driving force of the leader's focus. Values-focused leaders see problems or challenges in the clinical environment and seek to address them by leading as role models, being approachable and transparent so that others can bring issues to them. They lead by allowing others to see their confidence (in their own skills and knowledge), and they motivate their colleagues and demonstrate an empowered "can-do" attitude. They maintain support for their colleagues, and they maintain integrity while communicating effectively with their team or colleagues. Most significantly they are there in practice, not leading from above but from within facing the same issues, challenges and trials as their colleagues.

Values-based leaders (congruent leaders, authentic leaders, servant leaders, compassionate leaders, and others) listen when problems arise, or even identify them themselves (James et al. 2021a). They understand that solutions are best identified from within the team, within the cohort of healthcare staff at the coalface, who have experience of the issues and potential solutions to their concerns. Values-focused leaders have first-hand insights into the challenges and can empathise with the issues faced by staff and patients. Finally, values-focused leaders can stimulate debate, help with solutions and gather resources and information to address the issues at hand. The values-focused leader may not solve the problems themselves, but they may know a "man who can" (or woman) or have access to resources or others who can bring a resolution to the issue. Values-focused leaders bring a collective oversight to the challenge; the focus is on people, the skills or knowledge needed, the problem and the impact it is having on the core work of being able to effectively impact upon the organisation's values and not just an economic or managerially imposed change.

5.7 Summary

Organisations reflect the dynamics of small (and sometimes large) communities and working within them requires considerable skill. There are champions and heroes, cynics and naysayers. Change, no matter how positive, has the power to promote feelings of stress, anxiety, anger, hope, liberation and indifference, and whatever the change being proposed, managing it and dealing with the inevitable resistance will be central to the clinical leader's role and function.

It is clear that for the health service and care practices to improve, nurse leaders and health professionals need to be able to recognise what does not work well and develop strategies and solutions to change care practices, attitudes, systems and processes. This is relevant to clinical leadership practices because service improvement and developing the health service are based on effective change and innovation, and leadership is central to bringing about and facilitating these, with clinical leaders often in the role of "change champion" (Hendy 2012).

A range of tools for effectively managing change have been considered. These tools include strengths/weaknesses/opportunities/threats (SWOT) analysis; stakeholder analysis; Pettigrew's context/content/process model; the change management iceberg; PEST; nominal group technique; process re-engineering; FFA and other lesser approaches to managing change. Learning to employ change management approaches reduces a haphazard approach to change and innovation and offers nurses and other health professionals an opportunity to make a genuine impact on change in a planned, measured and strategic way.

Congruent leadership specifically indicates that leaders include everything they know and the knowledge of others, as well as all the resources that can be mustered, including their colleagues. A key leadership responsibility is participation in applying their care-focused values to encourage diversity and involvement from across the team, including other professional groups (Stanley 2008, 2019) and including the application of effective team working skills, covered in the following chapter.

6

Leadership and Teams

6.1 Introduction

This chapter will explore leadership and its role in the support of teams and team working. Leadership is not a solo activity, and many skills are required for leaders to deal with team development and task completion such as motivation, conflict resolution, clinical decision-making, innovation and addressing change. Leaders who are successful gain a personal insight and grasp of their own values and beliefs, their personal strengths, and weaknesses and how to marshal their team's strengths. Indeed, the leaders' capacity to recognise the strengths and limitations of their team and how to build, develop or maintain effective teams is vital.

In modern healthcare environments, ideal teams are rare. The reality is that teams commonly struggle to maintain success (Lencioni 2002; Cantwell 2015). They may appear cohesive but are often made up of people who are unsupportive, uncooperative and in competition, have personal grudges and are in open conflict, and as a result, talented, skilled people, frustrated by the limitations of a poorly performing team with poor leadership, fail to deliver their best work.

Team working can be very difficult to get right and although challenging to achieve, team working remains one of the best ways to organise people and tasks (Lencioni 2002; Pedler et al. 2004; Kalisch et al. 2010; Marlow et al. 2016). Falcone et al. (2008), Capella et al. (2010), Siassakos et al. (2011), Deering et al. (2011) and Steinemann et al. (2011), support Borrill et al. (2000, p. 371) who suggests that "*good teamwork can make a critical*

Notes On... Nursing Leadership, First Edition. Alison H. James and David Stanley.
© 2024 John Wiley & Sons Ltd. Published 2024 by John Wiley & Sons Ltd.

contribution to effectiveness and innovation in health care delivery and contributes to team members' well-being'."

The ability to work in teams is highly prized as a valuable organisational asset and team working feels right because this is what we have grown up with in our educational systems, sports clubs and early life experiences. Indeed, team working is a feature of our deep history with teams used in hunting and conflict representing our cultural development for millennia.

Effective team working is also identified as a requirement for enhanced clinical outcomes (Leggat 2007; Lyons and Popejoy 2014) and recognising the need for team working skills is particularly important in an organisation where "customer" service is important (Handy 1999). This is because often teams can make the best local decisions and are becoming largely self-managing (Elloy 2008). Organisations where teams work well have a common purpose, a culture of trust, support, interdependence and collaboration.

This chapter considers why team working matters from a nursing perspective, considers the value of support and challenge in helping teams work well and provides an overview of effective and ineffective teams and the role of a leader in managing conflict.

6.2 Healthcare Teams Defined

The World Health Organization (WHO 1988, p. 6) defined a healthcare team and teamwork in the following way:

> **Health team:** A group of people who share a common health goal and common objectives, determined by common needs, to the achievement of which each member of the team contributes, in accordance with his or her competence and skill, and in coordination with the functions of others. The manner and degree of such cooperation will vary and has to be determined by each society according to its own needs and resources. There can be no universally applicable composition of the health team.

While dated this definition indicates that there is no clear one way to define a healthcare team, and it alludes to the goal of creating greater inter-professional interaction within healthcare teams. Stanton and Chapman (2010) add that teams achieve their best through interdependent collaboration, open communication and shared decision-making, and they add that the notion of working in teams, within healthcare, instinctively feels good and particularly so in relation to a multidisciplinary and patient-focused context.

As ideal as teams may be, it is also clear that getting teamwork right can be difficult or challenging. Frequently team members are not supported, ill-coordinated and uncooperative, lack open, honest or collegial relationships and fail to work well to build cooperation or complete tasks successfully. Teams are not always needed, as some tasks can be done through good allocation of work to individuals or carried out by a group working more or less cooperatively (Lessard et al. 2008).

Teams are not really needed if the task relates to a simple exchange of information, if it involves simply sharing out work, updating each other and/or making simple operational decisions. These interactions relate mainly to reference and consultation groups with low levels of interaction, requiring only clear lines of communication (Lessard et al. 2008).

Teams are needed if the work is uncertain, difficult and complex, or where a high degree of collaboration and interdependence is required (Casey 1993; Stanley and Stanley 2018).

6.2.1 A Group

A **group** is defined as a number of individuals assembled together or having some unifying relationship (e.g. members of a club). These are groups because all the various members are related in some way to one another because of their involvement in a certain endeavour.

6.2.2 A Team

A **team** is described as a number of people associated together in specific work or activity. Parker (1990) indicates that a team is based on a highly interdependent set of people that:

- has defined goals and objectives (Markiewicz and West 2011),
- has an ongoing relationship and
- is focused on accomplishing a task.

Added to this are the ideas that teams work best if they recognise the value of:

- effective communication (Vogelsmeier and Scott-Cawiezell 2009),
- a singleness of mission,
- a willingness to cooperate and
- a commitment to each other.

The attributes of effective teams include the following:

- clarity of purpose/shared objectives or goals (Markiewicz and West 2011)
- informality
- participation
- diversity of styles/life experiences/thought (Leanne 2010)
- small to moderate size
- self-assessment and self-regulation
- meeting regularly
- interdependent working
- civilised disagreement
- consensus decisions
- clear roles and work assignments
- shared leadership
- listening

6.3 The Value of Teamwork

It is suggested that organisational culture has come to be seen as an important factor in the adaptability and performance of healthcare institutions (Meterko et al. 2004; Creighton and Smart 2022). Moreover, the degree of emphasis placed on teamwork and collaboration appears to be a pivotal dimension of organisational culture; for example, studies have shown that hospitals with a culture emphasising teamwork were able to further advance in their efforts to implement quality improvement processes (Shortell et al. 1995; Rathert and Fleming 2008; Hood et al. 2014; Stanley and Stanley 2018; Algunmeeyn et al. 2023). In another study of rehabilitation teams, Strasser et al. (2002) demonstrated that work cultures accentuating teamwork were associated with more effective rehabilitative professionals. In another study by Gifford et al. (2002), examining the obstetric units of seven hospitals found that an effective teamwork culture was associated with a lower turnover of nurses. It is also worth noting that teams construct their own internal culture and therefore occupy the position of a subculture within the larger culture of the organisation (Seago 1996). Understanding this and assessing team effectiveness can sometimes facilitate useful insights into the nature of team difficulties.

Understanding the connection between organisational cultures, with a focus on the value of teamwork, and improvements in a number of team performance indicators show that a strong relationship between patient satisfaction and a teamwork culture existed over other types of workplace culture (i.e. entrepreneurial, bureaucratic and rational) (Meterko et al. 2004; Creighton and Smart 2022; Indeed.com 2023), supporting the aim of the WHO (1988) to build workplace teams that enhanced patient satisfaction. There are a raft of studies that have focused on the benefits of inter-professional learning as a tool to facilitate greater attitudes towards teamwork in the clinical environment (Balmer et al. 2010; MacDonald et al. 2010; Newhouse and Spring 2010; Deering et al. 2011; Hood et al. 2014; Al-Sabei et al. 2022; Algunmeeyn et al. 2023), and it is clear that health professionals who learn together will find better ways to work and communicate with each other.

Jelphs and Dickinson (2008) and Markiewicz and West (2011) suggest that for a healthcare team to function effectively, it can only be accomplished with collaboration, interdependent working, effective communication and decision-making that is shared among the team members (including the clients). To achieve this, it requires several health professionals with complementary skills, common goals and the employment of a dynamic process to assess, plan and evaluate patient care (Creighton and Smart 2022).

They add that this approach to healthcare team working should result in better care and add value to organisational and staff-related outcomes (Jelphs and Dickinson 2008; Andersen et al. 2010; Kalisch and Lee 2010, 2013; Al-Sabei et al. 2022).

Reflective Activity 6.1

Before you read on… Consider these questions.

Do you work in a team?

Look at the attributes of an effective team described in this chapter. Does your team meet these attributes?

If not, what are the consequences for your workplace, the clients or patients and your own work satisfaction?

Leggat (2007) and Dawson et al. (2010) suggest the majority of healthcare workers work within team-based structures, but they may not work in effective teams. Healthcare teams could develop into pseudo-teams that are large, have a weak or non-existent requirement for interdependent working, fail to meet regularly and have few or no shared goals. Dawson et al. (2010) suggests that while 90% of NHS staff reported working in teams, less than 40% of them reported working in effective teams. If teams are to function well, they need the right mix of people with diverse skills, who communicate effectively, manage conflict well, and know and are all working towards common goals.

6.4 Types of Established Teams

Established teams usually fall into three or four basic sets. These are:

- High-Performance Teams,
- OK or Functional Teams,
- Struggling Teams and
- Self-Led Teams.

6.4.1 High-Performance Teams

These teams need little more than recognition and resourcing; they have established good working habits and address their own learning and development needs. They have "synergy" and an "all-hand" culture (Leanne 2010), with the rules for creating synergy related to:

- an established and clear purpose,
- active listening,
- compassionate inter-team behaviour (Rathert and Fleming 2008),
- truth-telling,
- being flexible,
- commitment to a resolution (agreeing to disagree, but moving on),
- high levels of passion and commitment,
- a sense that team members' perspectives and efforts are valued and
- a strong sense of "ownership" of the team/organisational goals/values (Guttman 2008, p. 35).

Rath and Conchie (2008) support these ideas and suggest that strong teams have these key attributes in common. These include a commitment to areas of their lives beyond the team, healthy debate within the team so that conflict is used positively and not avoided (Dunlap 2010; Leanne 2010), an eye for the big picture or organisational goals, and balancing their work and personal lives successfully. In addition, Rath and Conchie (2008) and Leanne (2010) propose that high-performance teams embrace diversity and act as magnets for talent, with their success acting as an attraction for other talented people. These suggestions were confirmed in a study by Rathert and Fleming (2008) who found that clinicians who perceived the ethical climate to be benevolent (supportive, encouraging and blame-free) had significantly greater teamwork in their teams. High-performance or effective teams also demonstrate effective team cohesion and greater focus on their common goal. Effective teams are also described as self-directing, having shared authority and decision-making and appearing leaderless at times. It has also been proposed that high-performing teams, where a climate of excellence already exists, use their excellence as a liberating force to support further innovation and generate a cycle of team interaction that leads to further excellence (Eisenbeiss et al. 2008).

While strong teams are desirable, they can have negative aspects too: becoming exclusive, complacent, competitive and big-headed, or they may lose sight of the big picture and focus on their own goals. They may build power through loyalty to the team and create barriers and competition with other teams to the detriment of the organisation, holding on to their own staff, stifling adaptability or innovation and rejecting newcomers. Thus, the balance between the potentially positive and the potentially negative issues need to be monitored carefully for success to be sustained.

6.4.2 OK or Functional Teams

These make up a large number of teams. Some may need no intervention while others need constant intervention to keep them functioning well. They might not work brilliantly, but they work well and have a competent balance. These teams may have tried and tested ways of addressing problems but lack the confidence to try new approaches. They are often based on traditional hierarchical structures with a traditional supervisor/subordinate relationship. They may have formal communication and authority lines, and these teams can be recognised right across the health service.

It is suggested that these sorts of teams are good at puzzles. These are made up of people with skills in the teams that know the way to find the answers. However, they may struggle with complex problems, lack confidence or struggle to create new partnerships and motivate each other, and fail to act collectively or collaboratively. Leadership in these teams is commonly shared, but members from a dominant professional group (such as medicine) may feel they have leadership authority (Sangvai et al. 2008; Cherry et al. 2010; Stanton et al. 2010), and some professionals may continue to focus on their own and not the overall team goals.

6.4.3 Struggling Teams

Struggling teams face the biggest challenges and may offer the closest reflection of a pseudo-team. They may fight turf wars within the team, have individuals that avoid work activities that will make them look bad, avoid disagreement and plain speaking, support "consensus" decisions that nobody wants and have poor-quality leadership, poor personal relationships and unresolved conflicts.

The main issue is often a lack of trust or commitment or as Algunmeeyn et al. (2023) identify there may also be issues with professionals misunderstanding other roles, or a lack of inter-professional socialisation or team working (Al-Sabei et al. 2022). Teams not committed to working together will not learn together and will often fail to develop. These teams lack a collective output, with Lencioni (2002) suggesting that there are five key areas evident in struggling teams. These are:

- absence of trust,
- fear of conflict,
- lack of commitment,
- avoidance of accountability and
- inattention to results.

Grenny (2010) adds that one reason teams may struggle is if they are "virtual" or if members are located in disparate sites. These sorts of teams are becoming more common in the business world and even in healthcare, with the advent of tele-health and other electronic media. To combat this Grenny (2010) recommends that even more effort is required to create team identity with a focus on mission, values and operating rules. In addition, communication skills need to be enhanced and supported, with greater social contacts established and fostered, motivation being monitored and rewarded appropriately and team performance being tracked on a daily or weekly basis.

If teams are not working well, it may be that the team as a whole is failing to function, or it may be that there are some pernicious individuals within the team that are – through bullying or controlling behaviour – bringing the contribution of the whole team down (Mikaelian and Stanley 2016). Assessing the core problems with struggling teams is vital before taking action, because if the issue is that of destructive individuals, reforming the team without addressing them will only transfer the problem to the newly created team, making its formation a more difficult process. Dubnicki (1991) developed an excellent team assessment questionnaire to facilitate a team's self-evaluation of their roles, activities, members' relationships and the work environment. Used correctly, this tool can be used to support an assessment of the success or otherwise of a team and identify areas where remedial action needs to be applied.

6.4.4 Self-Led Teams

These teams are often given a broad set of goals or objectives and then allowed to "get on with" the job of addressing them without the traditional manager or supervisor oversight. These "leaderless" teams are commonly referred to as self-led or self-managed teams. Of course, they are not "leaderless" as the leadership responsibilities are simply devolved to the team, so that the team assumes responsibility for its own systems, processes and "management" duties. In many respects, this is fulfilment of "followership" crossing over or amalgamating with leadership roles (Kellerman 2012; Raffo 2013; Malakyan 2014). Hurst et al. (2002) evaluated a set of integrated self-managed community health teams in the United Kingdom and found that these teams faced a number of barriers, including a loss of "corporateness" (associated with the previous structure) and poor communication processes as information struggled to cascade to the teams from "the top" of the organisation. However, the benefits were that teams enjoyed greater autonomy in decision-making, felt they had greater cohesion and felt that at a local "team" level the communication was more positive, and they undertook greater inter-professional sharing of health information and team working strategies (Hurst et al. 2002, p. 478). These benefits were supported by Stoker's (2007) study of leadership in self-managed teams, where flexible and supportive leadership styles were found to increase the effectiveness of individual team members and support an increase in team autonomy (Smama'h et al. 2023).

Self-led teams, sometimes referred to as "team leadership" (Jones and Bennett 2018), offer a "flat" structure (unlike the hierarchical structure of "traditional" teams and foster the engagement and participation of followers in the activity of leadership more easily) and the leadership approach required to support a self-managed team is also different with leaders in self-led teams needing to focus on trust building, effective communication, giving feedback, goal-setting activities, encouragement of innovation and decision-making (Elloy 2008). It should be noted that leaders operating within a team leadership model or in self-led or self-managed teams need to ensure trust, stability, compassion and hope to ensure that leaders can answer the question in this context of "why would anyone want to follow me?" Traditional teams required these factors to be addressed too, but in self-led teams these are the factors that appear to link directly to success and team effectiveness (Jones and Bennett 2018). Self-directed teams excel at using their team members' differences and sharing the team resources and assets to their overall advantage.

Reflective Activity 6.2

Before you read on... There are three/four basic types of teams described above (*high-performance teams, OK or functional teams, struggling teams, self-led teams*).

Which type of team do you think you work in?

Why is this?

What distinguishes you, as a team, from others?

How can you change the team's fortunes if needed?

6.5 Building Powerful Teams

There can be something liberating, even inspiring, about setting up a new team (MacDonald 2010). Clearly the objective aimed at will influence the make-up of the team, but in general terms, begin by selecting team members carefully. Look for team members and team leaders with sound innovation skills that can offer a diverse range of roles and ensure they can all be relied on from the outset. New teams should also be provided with a solid network of support and team cohesion should be fostered from the outset (MacDonald 2010). Creating new teams, while difficult and time-consuming, can often be very rewarding, because it avoids the sort of historical baggage that can interfere with working practices and allows communication channels and subcultures to develop as the new team does. In order to set up or create a new team, the following issues need to be considered:

- Clarify the purpose (objectives and goals) and task of the team (Hart 2010; MacDonald 2010).
- Establish and understand team roles (MacDonald et al. 2010).
- Create working processes and ground rules.
- Set up and run productive meetings.
- Make good decisions.
- Establish effective communication (Vogelsmeier and Scott-Cawiezell 2009; Dunlap 2010).
- Build the capacity of the team (Calendrillo 2009).
- Practise a reciprocal relationship whereby the leader and the led are able to influence each other (Zaccaro et al. 2001).
- Practise action learning.
- Keep all of these processes under review and
- Establish support and trust within the team (Dunlap 2010).

Tuckman (1965) suggested that teams go through the forming, storming, norming and performing stages that describe the basic reality taken to achieve team maturity (Pedler et al. 2004). Not allowing the time for teams to develop creates problems as teams are "thrown" together and are expected to be at their peak performance at once. The forming stage is vital and a too often neglected element of team building.

6.6 Support and Challenge

The key to getting teams to work well (and stay together) (Smama'h et al. 2023) is to build a balance between the two key issues of support and challenge (Iles 2011b).

6.6.1 Support

To ensure teams function well, teams need to feel supported (Ota et al. 2022; Smama'h et al. 2023). Nothing supports team members more than being listened to and feeling included or that they have a stake in the success and outcomes of the team. Thanking team members for their contribution and acknowledging their input are vital for team members to feel motivated to contribute further. Feedback is a key tool for team success, but it must be relevant, authentic, face to face if possible and timely (Iles 2011b; Ota et al. 2022).

6.6.2 Challenge

Kouzes and Posner (2010, p. 91) suggest that *"challenge is the crucible of greatness"* and that challenges act to bring people together, guide people through adversity, hardship and uncertainty. Nothing challenges more than opening the team members up to a good question or problem which makes them think about what they are trying to achieve and why (Handy 1999).

To build support and identify challenges, it is suggested that leaders:

- use customer surveys (staff, patients, user groups, colleagues),
- suggest potential issues that may lead to projects or challenges for the team to solve,
- use a facilitator from outside the team to act as a stimulus for discussion and debate,
- use action learning sets to focus the team on key issues and open dialog for suggestions and solutions,
- use a T, P, N (Total, Partial, Not at all) analysis approach,
- encourage team members to undertake self-analysis (such as Myers-Briggs Type analysis),
- have team members meet on a regular basis,

- tell the team when they have done a good job, praise the whole team and keep a record of their achievements (Balmer et al. 2010; Cantwell 2015) and
- set up a forum for discussion with open, honest conversation encouraged.

Iles (2011b) recommends three basic rules for dealing with team members to promote support and challenge. These are agreeing expectations, ensuring all team members have the skills needed to achieve the team outcomes and giving ongoing feedback when goals are met.

6.7 Team Building

Often when there are problems within a team, the proposed solution is to engage with "team building" in one form or another, and indeed, in healthcare environments strategies to improve teamwork commonly include team building or teamwork training (Dietz et al. 2014). Dyer (1987) and Dietz et al. (2014) suggested that team building and teamwork training can be enhanced by:

- setting the goals or priorities for the team,
- employing a team building/training framework,
- defining the parameters within which the team works,
- allocating or describing the way work is performed,
- considering the manner in which the team works: its processes, norms, decision-making and communication, and
- focusing upon the relationships among the people doing the work.

However, these approaches often generate only minor, short-lived improvements in morale and performance (Holland 2008) and are only of use after some sort of assessment has been undertaken to identify the teams' problem. There is also a view that team building can be a "bit of a laugh," avoiding the real "at work" issues. This perspective has grown from a number of "play-like" approaches to team building with paintball and other similar adventure activities used to build team spirit and cohesion. Another issue may be that the team seems to function well while away from the work environment during the team-building activity, but that old habits may prevail when back in the thick of a negative work culture that has not been addressed.

For team building and teamwork training (or indeed teamwork) to be successful, clear and present leadership is required (Holland 2008; Roh et al. 2020). When groups are struggling, effective leadership becomes even more important and so does understanding what matters to the team members. Leaders need to know, at least in part, what the problems are so they can avoid becoming defensive or simply window-dressing the problem. The advantage a clinical leader has is that they are often very much a part of the team and can support and facilitate better communication and more attention to problems and solutions.

6.8 Team Roles

For teams to work well, they need a variety of different people with a variety of skills and talents (Handy 1999; Frendsen 2014). Belbin (1981) undertook research into team roles that suggested the idea that a team made up of the brightest and best did not always produce the best results – this was called the Apollo syndrome. He also proposed, after considerable research, that successful teams are made up of people who fulfil a range of different roles, identifying eight (or nine) key team roles.

The result of the research was a questionnaire used to support teams to identify their "preferred" team role and to help teams gain an insight into their make-up and development needs. Belbin's (1981) approach to team role assessment offers a robust and highly effective insight into how teams work and represents an accurate approach to assessing individual behaviour and its impact on team function. In Belbin's words, *"Nobody is perfect . . . but a team can be."* Therefore, gaining an understanding of teams, how they are made up and individual team roles can be of great benefit for team success (Belbin 1981; Frendsen 2014). The eight key team roles described by Belbin (nine if the role of the "specialist" is counted) are as follows:

- **Plant**: introverted, but intellectually dominant. The source of original ideas and described as creative, imaginative and unorthodox.
- **Coordinator:** presides over the team and coordinates their efforts. Described as mature and confident and clarifies goals.
- **Monitor/evaluator:** intelligent and directed towards analytical rather than creative energies. Described as sober, strategic and an accurate judge.

- **Implementer:** turns ideas into manageable tasks. Schedules, charts and plans are their thing. Described as disciplined, reliable and a doer.
- **Completer/finisher:** checks details, and makes sure schedules are met, drives others on to complete their tasks. Described as painstaking and conscientious and delivers on time.
- **Resource investigator:** commonly a popular member of a team. Described as sociable, relaxed, extrovert and enthusiastic and develops contacts. Their role is to make or bring in new contacts, acting as a salesperson or liaison for the team.
- **Shaper:** described as highly strung, outgoing and dominant; can also be challenging, dynamic and courageous.
- **Team worker:** holds the team together, supporting others, listening, encouraging and acting as a link person for others. Described as diplomatic, mild and cooperative.
- **Specialist:** often called into teams for special knowledge or skills, frequently do not stay in the team beyond their immediate requirements. May be seen as single-minded.

The advantage of understanding team roles from Belbin's perspective is that the teams' needs will often dictate the most appropriate leader at the most relevant time so that no one role is specifically affiliated with team leadership. Therefore, different roles may be needed to different degrees at different times. For example, if a team is being formed, it may need a strong shaper or plant to motivate team members or generate ideas.

It is not essential that teams have eight people, each undertaking one of the eight Belbin roles, but teams do need people to be aware of these various roles and find ways to fulfil them. In small teams, people can assume more than one role, while in larger teams it would be reasonable to expect that different people undertake the same team role. Establishing team roles is also beneficial when it comes to team decision-making. At times, teams struggle to make effective decisions and having clear ground rules and clear team roles can facilitate confidence and allow teams to reach alignment with decision-making (Frisch 2008).

Seeing the variety of roles as described by Belbin (1981) implies that teams are made up of a variety of different people with different skills and that the most effective teams recognise this and act to include these various roles. Teams need all types, team workers, coordinators and finishers, to function well. This perspective is supported by Leggat (2007) who suggested that team working competencies were perceived to be different for management and clinical teams, further reinforcing the value of having different people with different skills populating teams. However, it should be remembered that in spite of having well-defined team roles, the interaction of people in teams and the impact of their personalities can – and often does – have an effect on team friction or relationships within the team. The key in these circumstances is to manage conflict constructively.

6.9 Leadership and Teams

As well as key attributes for teams to function, having effective leadership within the team is considered vital (Borrill et al. 2000; Lencioni 2002; Harkins 2008; Kalisch et al. 2010) and when building teams, it is even more essential. Team leaders are required to demonstrate their confidence in the team and themselves. Once fear sets in and confidence is eroded, the teams' belief in the leader falters and building or maintaining the team becomes very difficult. Harkins (2008) proposes there are three things team leaders should achieve in order to effectively lead a team:

1) Ensure the team goals are clearly defined.
2) Establish team roles so that team members are clear about the part they play in the team.
3) Team leaders should use language and role model actions to build trust (LaBrosse 2008), motivate others and build positive energy.

6.10 Trust

Achieving the three steps above sets team leaders apart as "*high-impact*" team leaders (Harkins 2008). Lencioni (2002) adds that leaders need to demonstrate genuine "vulnerability" as a way of building team trust. Feigned vulnerability can be seen as manipulation and will only destroy trust. In addition, leaders need to foster excellent conflict management and conflict resolution skills and be comfortable making decisions (Lencioni 2002). In Borrill et al.'s (2000) study, teams without effective leadership reported poor participation, a lack of clarity about objectives, lower commitment to quality and innovation and poor mental health among team members. Therefore, efficient team leadership leads to effective team processes, higher performance, greater innovation and greater staff satisfaction (Kalisch and Lee 2010) all leading to better teamwork (and better led teams), which leads to better performance and greater patient satisfaction (Siassakos et al. 2011).

Leaders are often people who care about people and this care translates into a willingness to focus time and energy on members of the team. From this perspective caring is risking being with the team and sharing both suffering and joy. Behaviours that demonstrate caring include giving of oneself in terms of warmth, passion and, particularly, giving one's time. The second aspect of caring is truly listening to team members, hearing and understanding them. The third aspect is being 100% present for them. The fourth is to honour the team members and to see their wholeness, their possibilities and their hope. Leading a team is one of the most difficult things to do, with Wageman et al. (2009) suggesting that a key leadership skill is the capability of team leaders to judge the time for action or analysis within the team. Knowing your values and that of the team members can help the team align and sometimes, we all need to be reminded, have a reset and refocus in the busy and complex day-to-day demands of healthcare.

Reflective Activity 6.3

Before you read on... Consider the priorities for your team and the individuals within it, and their need for individual development and team development.
Consider how you communicate your core values.
Are all the team members aware of these?
How do these align to the clinical area's philosophy and professional values?

Being a team member is also difficult because being part of a team is the same as being part of a relationship, and as with any other relationship in our lives – being in a team, building a team or leading a team – it involves risk and requires commitment, trust and character, both personal and professional. The team leader's role should be very much focused on sustaining the relationships needed for the team to be effective (Calendrillo 2009). Crosbie (2006) found that failing to provide effective leadership diminished autonomy and resulted in a lack of inclusiveness in decision-making, which impacted negatively on team members' job satisfaction. Other key factors impacted when leaders employed control or a hierarchical structure in the team, or when leaders fail to demonstrate appreciation for team members, offered favouritism to some team members, failed to offer direction, and were poor decision-makers or failed to demonstrate caring or trust towards their teams.

Health professionals are increasingly to be found working in interprofessional teams. However, if different professional groups are to genuinely employ team working in the clinical setting, training and education need to focus specifically on the skills and attributes of team cohesion (Guise and Segel 2008; Andersen et al. 2010; Capella et al. 2010; Siassakos et al. 2011; Steinemann et al. 2011). Learning about teams will not come from just being in one, and considerable benefits for quality improvement, innovation and patient safety will flow from attention to enhanced leadership and teamwork insights in undergraduate programs. Teams do not always work in all situations; they can sometimes stifle dissent and creativity. However, they can produce powerful groups of people who need little direct management and often appear to be "leaderless." In some regard, teams are becoming the new management.

Teams offer hope to all. For even if your performance is mediocre or if you feel insignificant, you can do great things as part of a team. You are needed in a team.

6.11 Summary

This chapter has outlined that teams don't always work in all situations, that teams and groups are different and that effective teams have a clear purpose and informality; meet regularly; have interdependent working, civilised disagreement, consensus decisions, shared leadership and a diversity of styles; are usually small to moderate in size; and employ self-assessment and self-regulation. Sometimes effective teams can produce powerful outcomes, without the need for direction and may even appear "leaderless." It is proposed that there are three or four basic types of teams: high-performance, OK or functional, struggling teams and self-managed or self-led teams. Creating new teams requires considerable time and clarity of purpose, the establishment of team roles, clear working processes and ground rules, clear decisions, effective communication and the establishment of support and trust. Effective teams also have several different roles that team members can take within them to make the team function effectively. These are the plant, coordinator, monitor/evaluator, implementer, completer/finisher, resource investigator, shaper, team worker and, in some circumstances, specialist. Successful teams have a clear balance between support and challenge and manage to see the advantage of a variety of people, undertaking different roles to offer strength and diversity. Team leaders support teams by caring about team members, by listening to them, giving of their time and being present. These are expressed as trust in the team.

7

Leadership and Networking

7.1   Introduction

This chapter has nothing to do with fishing . . . or does it? As it will address the important leadership skill of networking. Personal, professional, organisational, strategic and even international networks are central for effective leadership to flourish. Networking can be defined as an interconnected system of things or people. These are often informal or, can sometimes be formal (Marquis and Huston 2021) and relate to an exchange of information or services among individuals, groups or institutions, specifically the cultivation of productive relationships for employment or business. More recently networking is associated with information technology (IT) and the development of social networks in reference to the interconnection of computers.

However, networks are also associations between individuals or groups of people where the association can be personal relationships, relationships in industry, in a sporting context, in entertainment, in a business context, as part of a professional relationship or through clients and customers, and encountered in the course of your professional activities. Indeed, they can be relationships with anyone. Opportunities for networking happen whenever people meet, and, in many respects, networking is about how things get done (Drake 2017).

Notes On... Nursing Leadership, First Edition. Alison H. James and David Stanley.
© 2024 John Wiley & Sons Ltd. Published 2024 by John Wiley & Sons Ltd.

7.2   Networking and Influencing for Change

Bresnen (2017, p. 140) suggests the primary purpose of networking is to acquire or share knowledge, followed by networking for support, such as *"emotional reassurance, personal validation, consolation or the expression of feelings outside of the immediate work context."* The role of networking for career advancement is also through connecting with new opportunities and is useful to secure influence over decision-making and desired behaviours or actions. Marquis and Huston (2021) suggest that networking increases power and influence by forming alliances with peers, senior and junior co-workers, and colleagues outside the organisation.

Establishing effective networks is an essential aspect of a leader's role, particularly if formal power is not an option. Networking gives a leader access to contacts, information, resources and support so that they can accomplish a host of tasks, employ creativity and offer innovative solutions to problems. Networking adds collective wisdom and influence for leaders to gain greater support, adding a vital source of knowledge, energy and information on current or future events within an organisation and in wider health professional associations.

7.3   The Skills of Networking

Becoming an effective networker can be achieved with a minimal amount of effort; however, fostering a specific network for a specific purpose may take a degree of attention and focus and require some thought to set up. Although networking may not come naturally to some people, being a good networker by simply interacting and exchanging ideas can be an easy thing to achieve (Kaweckyj 2019).

To enhance effective networking and build effective relationships with the people with whom you connect, remember that first impressions count, whether face to face or online. Look for opportunities when you meet people online through professional discussion groups or at conferences or meetings. Experienced health professionals will use networking to extend their influence by meeting new colleagues. Think about extending your network to include health professionals from a range of disciplines and at various stages of their professional careers. New starters can bring fresh perspectives; experienced colleagues can provide a wealth of information (Prado et al. 2020). Here are some tips for establishing effective networks or developing professional networking skills.

- **Extend Your Profile** – successful networking requires you to find people with whom you want to be known (Kaweckyj 2019).
- **Use Social Networks** – a detailed social media profile can be beneficial and may support your ongoing career goals. Pizzuti et al. (2020) in their study of healthcare workers (nurses, pharmacists, administrators and doctors) believe that social media is an effective tool for healthcare education. However, keep your professional profile separate from your social activities and be aware of the risks and exposure social media can present.
- **Engage with Professional Development** – completing a course and acquiring more information is an excellent way to learn more and meet new people who have similar interests.
- **Go to Conferences** – conferences play a critical role in the professional development of health professionals and provide many opportunities to network and build relationships (Lindsay 2018). However, they can be costly, so explore sources of funding and opportunities for presenting.
- **Volunteering and Citizenship** – this simply means making yourself available for community-focused tasks bringing you into more contact with others and contributing to the benefit of the community.
- **Join a Professional Organisation** – membership of professional organisations can bring credibility, keep you current with best practices and give you access to a voice for effecting changes in subjects that interest you.
- **Look Beyond Your Own Organisation** – your networks are richer if they stretch beyond your workplace and even beyond one organisation. Extend your view to what is happening globally in healthcare and nursing.
- **Be Professionally Committed and Have Clear Messages** – leadership requires clear communication. Develop a professional profile and be clear what your interest and specialist area is. This will allow others to identify your area of interest and increase opportunities for networking.
- **Join Professional Discussion Groups** – professional organisations and online discussion groups often function within a social networking

context and include forums and chat rooms to engender interactions and ideas and encourage collaborative practice. This can have global reach and extend opportunities.

- **Mentor or Coach Others or Be Mentored/Coached** – being a mentor or coach or seeking out and engaging with a mentor/coach for yourself can enhance your leadership and learning skills and show your commitment and support for others (Houston 2020).
- **Travel (for professional reasons)** – a radical way to widen your networks is actually to go and work in other countries and locations. This can extend your professional practice and experience and lead to lifelong networks.
- **Develop a Clinical Supervision Process** – clinical supervision has a focus on progressing the professionals' reflective skills on clinical practice and competence with the support and guidance of a more experienced professional to enhance accountability and patient safety in complex situations (King et al. 2020; Martin and Snowdon 2020).
- **Expand Your Informal "Coffee" Network** – health professionals often meet over coffee or tea, and making an effort to have informal social meetings with professionals from other areas or departments will significantly expand your professional network and give you access to information from other parts of the organisation.
- **Publish** – published work enters the global network of professional work, enriching others' knowledge and allowing them to recognise your professional contribution. It may seem daunting to begin with; however, there are many supportive opportunities. Professional journals often offer online writing hints and tips or courses. Approach authors in your field of interest and ask to discuss ideas for publication.
- **Be Genuine and Authentic** – so that you can build trust in your relationships, being clear about your goals when you network so that you can focus on the right networks, connecting with groups and interests that spark your interest and attention. Listen and ask open-ended questions in networking conversations, become known as a powerful or useful resource for others, regularly follow up on the contacts you have made, and be clear about how you can be of help to others, rather than just focusing on what the network can do for you.

- **Use LinkedIn** – as a professional social network, LinkedIn is gaining ground. Established in 2003, it now has over 400 million users worldwide (Higgs et al. 2019).
- **Use Other Social Media Platforms** – such as Facebook, Twitter, YouTube, Instagram, WhatsApp, Snapchat, Reddit, "X" and Pinterest. Through the use of social media, reaching out to people far beyond your everyday contacts is beneficial, although remember that social media networks are a tool and are incredibly valuable, but only when used appropriately and wisely as social media platforms come with their own inbuilt risks (see Box 7.1 below).

> Networking is not a sin, cast your net, see what comes in.

Box 7.1   The Dangers and Risks of Social Media Use

There are several serious risks with the use of social media platforms. While the ability to link with potentially millions of people all over the world on a host of issues seems like a wonderful opportunity, social media platforms are not designed with users' interests at heart. Instead, they are specifically designed to promote ongoing use of the platform, offering "click-bait" for users to follow, leading to the potential to feed preconceived ideas and take users down rabbit holes that take them to other often biased sites and ideas.

The underlying business model of Google and Facebook, and other platforms, is to harvest and monetise our personal information. This model's fundamental characteristic is to aggregate vast amounts of data on people by keeping them on the platforms for as long as possible, use that data to build incredibly detailed profiles on people's lives and behaviour, and monetise it by selling data to whoever wants to influence the user (https://www.amnesty. org.au/the-social-dilemma-2/?cn=trd&mc=click&pli=23501504& PluID=0&ord={timestamp}&gclid=EAIaIQobChMIqKumusjL_ wIVaZhmAh2lOAZMEAAYAyAAEgKew_D_BwE).

The aim of social media platforms is basically user surveillance and this is not only inherently incompatible with the right to privacy, but poses a systemic threat to a range of other rights including freedom of opinion and expression, freedom of thought and the right to equality and non-discrimination (https://www.amnesty.org/en/documents/pol30/1404/2019/en/). These platforms use algorithms to determine the content on our feeds and the ads that will be served to us. Very often these algorithms amplify disinformation and divisive content, fuel racism and hate speech and influence our own beliefs and opinions.

7.4 Summary

Being an effective leader means using your own skills and abilities and those of the people around you. The net effect is one of synergy where the sum of the parts is greater than the whole. There are specific skills and ways to build networks and although care should be taken when applying the gifts of social media networks, they may offer a speedy way to link with likeminded colleagues and nurses from other parts of the world.

8

Leadership and Values

8.1   Introduction

This chapter will explore the importance of values-based approaches to nursing leadership. The relationship between professional values and approaches to leadership will be addressed and how this can influence others in areas such as role modelling and experience. How nursing leadership is perceived is introduced along with considerations for the importance of values-based nursing leadership for power balance and social justice.

Nurses and professional healthcare practitioners align themselves to the professional values of their chosen profession and indeed, with regulation, comes the expectation and requirement that those values will be central to the decision-making and actions carried out in their day-to-day practice. We know that when considering self-leadership, student nurses look to mentors and role models and their experience of leadership can have an impact on how they view leadership (James et al. 2022). Bruner (1986) explains that in communities of practice where values, knowledge and cultures are shared, such as nursing, "critical events" or experiences which alter perceptions can have a profound impact. James (2020) explored "critical events," experiences of leadership which impact individuals, both in a positive and negative way, and shape views of leadership. When a nurse leader demonstrates professional values in practice, as Stanley (2019) outlines in the development of the congruent leadership theory, it is clear that the attributes align to nursing principles such as treating everyone with dignity and respect and demonstrating integrity. However, it is also evident

Notes On... Nursing Leadership, First Edition. Alison H. James and David Stanley.
© 2024 John Wiley & Sons Ltd. Published 2024 by John Wiley & Sons Ltd.

that instances of incivility and bullying are also an issue in nursing with studies suggesting it is 10–15% higher in nursing than in other occupations (Hunt and Marini 2012). Clearly these actions are not aligned to the professional values of nursing and pose a danger to less experienced nurses, in establishing incivility as an accepted practice on which to base professional behaviours.

Demonstrations of incivility and bullying have been linked to oppressed groups, lacking in self-esteem and power (Roberts 2015; Mikaelian and Stanley 2016; James and Bennett 2022a). As individuals within such a group nurse leaders may also be susceptible to such behaviour, directing frustrations on their own peers. Therefore, within this chapter we consider what can be done to ensure leadership in nursing remains values based and to ensure incivility is not tolerated. When faced with challenges of power and conflict, how can leaders maintain professional integrity and ensure their actions and behaviours remain aligned.

> Values are the glue that binds a team; core values also drive our purpose.

8.2 Change and Values

> Open your arms to change but don't let go of your values.
> Dalai Lama (2000)

We discussed in Chapter 5 how leaders can influence change and innovation. Here we deal with change on an individual level. As people develop and gain experience, they may change in their thinking and approach to things. That is perhaps a natural progression of our human development. Learning comes from errors and mistakes, from others (role models) and from gaining different experiences and learning. These are known as:

- tacit knowledge: gained from personal experience,
- explicit knowledge: knowledge which is documented, easy to share and write down, and
- implicit knowledge: application of explicit knowledge such as transferable skills.

All of these types of learning and development are important for nurse leaders to progress and develop. However, because of the complexities, hierarchies and cultural structures of healthcare organisations, the values and learning can be forgotten or swayed, which can result in failures of leadership (James and Bennett 2022b). Rather than empower colleagues and the profession, disempowerment and self-destruction can be the result, causing damage to the fragility of nursing's strength as a profession of integrity. When individual leaders lose sight of core values and become distracted or indeed perhaps feel powerless against more powerful influencers, cultures of negativity and neglect can flourish. When leadership fails to be values focused, human focused, transparent in its decision-making, open to questioning and self-reflective. Negative cultures and ultimately unsafe environments can emerge, as documented in recent examples in the United Kingdom, such as the Francis Report (2013) and more recently in the Ockenden Review (2022).

Kaiser (2017) found that behaviours of nursing leaders that resulted in adverse impacts on staff were:

- not encouraging staff to be involved in decision-making,
- being distant and remote and lacking in relationship forming with staff,
- being controlling and authoritarian,
- not being visible and present in clinical areas and
- not encouraging staff to be involved in wider decisions.

Leaders who do not address incivility or allow competitiveness and adversarial attitudes do not address the issues of drift from professional values, and it is suggested that when staff perceive a lack of response and action to incivility, it can become the accepted and normalised behaviour (Clark et al. 2013). While we attribute leadership as being possible for all nurses, with no attachment to position or role, it must be acknowledged that in our healthcare systems, leadership can be associated with position and progression, or climbing the career ladder. In some situations, this results in distancing from clinical practice to a focus on management. This personal change can perhaps induce a feeling of remoteness from the clinical day-to-day professional challenges of providing quality patient care and move to complex management decision-making of higher level and macro-organisation needs. It is clear from the reports mentioned earlier, a constant reminder that the nature and principles of nursing are for the benefit of patients. So keeping professional values at the fore are a priority for nurse leaders whatever positional role they acquire and managing incivility and negative cultures are important to maintain these.

Kelly et al. (2023) in their study of Executive Nurse Directors (these are nurses who hold strategic- and operational-level leadership in hospitals in the United Kingdom, other titles are used globally) found that while they are expected to be visible and present in clinical areas and to staff, some felt low self-esteem and professionally vulnerable. Therefore, career progression to high-level leadership and management roles can perhaps be distancing and challenging. Maintaining professional values and clearly communicating these to others means nurse leaders may thrive at any positional level and importantly set the culture and expectations of respect for patients and colleagues, transparency and openness of responsibility, being patient centred and knowledgeable, and demonstrating values-based professionalism within their organisations.

8.3 Facing the Challenges and Balancing Power

Whether leaders are clinically positioned or at executive level, the relevance of power will often be of consequence as both politics and power are central to the provision and delivery of healthcare globally. Whether through national or local policy, nurses must be aware of and manage the influence of these forces as they can directly impact the allocation of resources, the effectiveness of provision and the equity of healthcare. Locally, we know that power balances inhabit our workplaces, our professions and our teams, and they can be positive and negative influences. Being aware of these can help navigate the challenging situations and decision-making a nurse leader may be faced with and provide a broader view of what the issues really are (James and Bennett 2022a). It is helpful to know that there are different types of power sources which Yoder-Wise (2015) explores and provides examples such as:

- **Resource power** – controlling of allocation of resources and budgets, promotion opportunities, reward and withholding reward.
- **Information power** – having access to information or knowledge and controlling the sharing or withholding.

- **Expert power** – from knowledge or expertise that has value.
- **Coercive power** – the generation of fear by threat.
- **Charismatic power** – the ability to be accepted by others and connection with others in authority.
- **Legitimate power** – having a titled position which provides authority.
- **Reward power** – the ability to grant awards or reward which is valued by others.

Being aware of these types of power enables us to realise it is not negative or indeed positive in itself, rather how it used and to what purpose. As a nurse leader it is possible to apply the use of power to great effect when the purpose and desired outcome is aligned to professional values.

Unfortunately, within large organisations, people may well feel powerlessness, or lack of control, over their work environment. Nurse leaders who wish others and their teams to thrive can enable feelings of power by engaging them in decision-making, seeking out their opinions and views and acting on these in a demonstrative way, placing value on their insights (James and Bennett 2022a).

Nurse leaders are considered as influencing, whether it is about decisions about patient care or within a team discussion, or indeed wider. Using influence involves managing power, and how you apply this will depend on your values, on your professional approach, on your leadership approach and on your determination and conviction. It may be that you need to advocate for a patient, are involved in a discussion of resource priorities or are advocating for another member of staff. The way you apply your influencing power is something that takes time and experience to master, but being aware of where values feature in this is important. When values leave the equation, power can be used negatively or for pure personal gain.

Consider the following types of influencing styles (Stanley et al. 2023), and how you might apply these with your own approach to leadership while keeping your professional values at the centre:

- **Assertive persuasion** – influencing through the weight of your argument, a logical approach using reasoning.
- **Reward and punishment** – use of bargaining, incentivising and reward for compliance, while withdrawing these in an attempt to control, or as punishment for non-compliance.

- **Participation and trust** – instilling trust through engagement, listening and transparency about own vulnerabilities.
- **Common vision** – agreeing on a collective vision for the future with clear communication and conviction to enable buy in from others.
- **Common values** – the leader may demonstrate their values through actions, associations with professions and symbolism. A congruent leader may align to this as actions convey their values base.

> The real challenge for nurse leaders is to remain true to their core values while holding onto their humanity in the face of a rapidly changing world.

8.4 Leadership and Its Role in Social Justice

The recent challenges of the COVID-19 pandemic have brought to focus the relationship between socioeconomic and political influences on healthcare in all societies. These aspects clearly influence the allocation of resources and delivery of services (James et al. 2021b). As a values-based profession which aims to provide a caring service for the population, the association to fairness of access and equality are central to nursing principles. However, it is challenging for many nurses to believe they are able to influence such wide and powerful forces. Being aware of critical social theory can provide the clinical nurse leader with a wider consciousness and while it is sometimes easier to deal day to day with the local challenges of the role, being outward facing and aware can allow leaders to challenge decisions, assumptions and inequality.

Nursing and healthcare are entangled with social justice principles because of the values and ethical principles on which they are founded. Fairness, justice and equality are central principles for the clinical leader, however the challenge of corporate organisational decision-making and wider political directives can be a source of tension if these affect patient care. Through enlightenment, empowerment, humanity and emancipation, clinical leaders can engage with social justice and move their influence forward (Fay 1987; James et al. 2021b).

Reflective Activity 8.1

Before you read on ... Consider the three-phase process of enlightenment, empowerment and emancipation (Fay 1987).

Enlightenment can mean the ability of a group (nurses in this instance) to view themselves in a different way. With empowerment, this can lead to emancipation.

How might nurses change society's view of the profession to benefit their influence on decision-making at higher levels of power?

8.5 Summary

This chapter has explored the importance of values-based approaches to nursing leadership and how power, politics and social justice are relevant and may influence and challenge nurse leaders. Being aware of influencing styles and power sources can equip leaders with identifying how others may use them and how to apply them. Balancing this and developing a wider consciousness of wider influences can provide the nurse leader with greater depth of analysis of issues and innovative approaches to having a voice and ensuring ethical principles remain a focus in healthcare.

9

The Challenges of Nurse Leadership

9.1 Introduction

This chapter will focus on the challenges of leadership and the importance of the leader's well-being. In recent years, leaders in healthcare have experienced extreme challenges, and this chapter will explore the risks and effects of leading during a crisis. Much research has been published during and after the COVID-19 pandemic, building on the dearth of knowledge in this area pre-pandemic, and this has brought suggestions of strategies for leading. It has also identified gaps in preparation and a realisation that while both our healthcare systems and individuals within may cope with short episodes of high impact, the long-term and unpredictable nature of COVID-19 caused an immense strain and uncertainty and continues to do so.

The COVID-19 pandemic has introduced a new range of vocabulary and in some countries, nurse leaders have had to quickly grasp their meaning to explain and relate their importance to patients and staff, such as "lockdown," "self-isolation," "pandemic," "endemic" and the language of political leaders who use military metaphors of war. Using this terminology may have been an attempt to unify communities and to ensure the seriousness of the situation was realised. However, it also had the effect of instilling fear for control and compliance. For nurses working with patients' day to day, fear was another issue to deal with in caring for patients with health needs while also in great fear of being infected themselves. Linguistic creativity is often used in times of serious social

Notes On... Nursing Leadership, First Edition. Alison H. James and David Stanley.
© 2024 John Wiley & Sons Ltd. Published 2024 by John Wiley & Sons Ltd.

crisis and is not new (Flusberg et al. 2018). However, as a nurse leader during a crisis, care and the application of emotional intelligence is needed to be aware of the impact of how information is communicated, how it is received and the reaction to messages from perceived healthcare leaders and their followers.

The image of nursing during the pandemic has varied, from "*angelic tropes*" to "*vexatious protestors*" as explored by Bennett et al. (2020) at the height of the pandemic and again as the COVID-19 pandemic waned (James et al. 2023). This is challenging for nurse leaders as historically nursing has been viewed as symbolic of servitude and the nature and needs of the profession have changed. Nurse leaders are more than able, skilled and knowledgeable to have an influencing voice in the decisions of healthcare policy; yet for some, this remains a challenge. Looking forward, nurse leaders have considerable power to continue to lobby for the profession, using learning from challenges to build the presence of nursing on the global stage.

9.2 Leading During Challenging Times

> There is a crack in everything. That's how the light gets in.
> Leonard Cohen (2014, p. 366)

While the experience of nurses during the pandemic has often been traumatic and challenging, there are undoubtedly opportunities to learn and prepare for the future. In order to do that, there is a need for transparency and open discussions which confront difficult issues. It can be argued that decisions had to be made and the "command and control" approach of many governments was needed. Difficult decisions and rapid actions were required, often stepping into the unknown of what the future held. Nurse leaders, alongside other health professionals, were required to act on many of these decisions and make decisions on the clinical floor, and there is much written now on the issues of moral injury and moral distress; the emotional response following events that contradict or violate a person's ethical or moral stance (Litz et al. 2009). Frei and Morriss (2020) and Thompson and Kusy (2021) agree that teams who are able to maintain unity and interconnection demonstrate honesty and trust, authenticity and empathy, and these are often set and directed by the nurse leader in a clinical context. Worline and Dutton (2017) suggest social connection and altruism are linked to compassion and empathy and having core professional values can improve unity in teams. More than ever, during challenging times, a compassionate and congruent leader can encourage cohesion and empathy within a team, ensuring that even during the most difficult times, a team can feel trusted, listened to and supported. Allowing the expression of emotions and indeed, being courageous by demonstrating their own emotions, clinical leaders can place value on the experiences and impact of their co-workers and provide reassurance (Thompson and Kusy 2021).

9.3   Examples of Leading Through Crises

Learning from leadership examples outside of healthcare can allow us to gain a wide perspective on how people manage adversity well. There will be examples perhaps locally and within your organisation that can inspire and motivate, and it is good to share these examples for staff. Meanwhile we can look wider, and below are some examples of leaders and their approaches to crisis leadership, which have provided positive cases for effective leadership approaches.

1) **Decisive action with displayed compassion:** Jacinda Ardern - former Prime Minister, New Zealand.

   Applying an approach of decisive action, clear communication and expression of humanity, Jacinda Ardern limited deaths related to COVID-19 to far fewer than many countries and eased lockdown controls earlier. With prior experience in dealing with tragic events, she demonstrated openly her sensitivity and compassion, bringing people together and making swift policy changes to gun laws.

2) **Giving followers direction and roles recognising their value, instilling trust:** Earnest Shackleton - Explorer and Captain of *Endurance*.

   In 1915 *Endurance*, Shackleton's ship, became stuck in the ice on an exploration to the Antarctic. Shackleton realised that he and his crew would have to wait out the brutal weather conditions trapped in ice. To keep the crew's morale high he insisted each man maintain duties, keeping daily routines and tasks, establishing order and keeping his men focused in uncertain times that were filled with danger. Shackleton responded to changing circumstances. When the ship was no longer habitable, crushed by the ice, he instructed his men to build a camp on the ice. Moving the crew on, not really knowing the outcome, he reached an uninhabited island. Knowing that no one knew if they were alive and therefore with no chance of rescue, he identified a group of men to accompany him in one of the three lifeboats 800 miles to find help. Four months and three unsuccessful rescue attempts later, Shackleton arrived back to rescue the rest of his team. They were all alive.

Reflective Activity 9.1

Before you read on … Consider the approaches taken by the examples of leadership above.

Think of other examples of leadership you may have read about or seen in practice. What other leadership attributes can you add that made these examples memorable and effective, which were particularly relevant to a time of crisis?

9.4 Leading with Self-Care

The very nature of a crisis leaves an indelible effect on those who are involved in leadership during its process (see Chapter 4). The effects may present as exhaustion and burnout from the intensity of work and decision-making; it may be grief from losing patients, staff or indeed loved ones. It is essential therefore to be aware of the effects on others and on yourself, and to respond to those as needed. Taking care of your own well-being is essential not only for you but also for those you work with and for those close to you. Being self-aware, you can identify when you are focused and effective, and when you are not. Therefore, as a leader, it is important to realise that others can observe these effects in you and may respond accordingly.

Stanley et al. (2023) suggest strategies for well-being which are listed here:

- Seek out opportunities to share your story and create a safe space and opportunities for others to share their stories. Expressing emotions and feelings can prevent fear and frustrations developing.
- Explore and access mindfulness techniques for your own development and that of the team.
- Create and support an environment of trust in the team to support and encourage innovation.
- Develop mentorship and encourage buddying for staff. Seek out coaching opportunities for your own development.
- Role model authentic and compassionate, values-based leadership.
- Prioritise recovery strategies and advocate for staff recovery time.
- Consider daily briefings if rapid change is evident to ensure clear communication.
- Encourage and involve staff in decision-making to develop ownership.
- Prioritise well-being for staff and advocate for staff and resources for self-care cultures.

9.5 Summary

Leading is not easy and doing so requires leaders to face a raft of challenges, including the following:

- Leading in times of crisis.
- Having to grasp new vocabulary.
- Having to deal with a more health literate or more information literate public (even if the information is incorrect or misguided).
- Leading with limited resources.
- Leading with limited support.
- Having their leadership role misunderstood (because of historical precedents).
- Leading in the face of moral and ethical distress.
- Leading in the face of adversity.
- Failing to grasp the value of self-care as a strategy for dealing with the leadership role.

Taking time for self-care is important for all nurse leaders, for your team and for the organisation as a whole. In the next chapter, "Followership" is explored and the importance of having positive followers for effective leadership is clearly of benefit to all (Grint 2000). For your own leadership to develop and for others to function effectively, prioritising well-being is important, especially during times of highly challenging demands and crisis.

10

Followership

10.1 Introduction

Hersey et al. (1996) suggest that "followership" is the flip side of leadership. Followers are described as vital because they accept or reject the leader and determine the leader's personal power (Alwazzan 2017). The interaction between followers and leaders is central because it occurs on a multitude of levels, and therefore followers should be considered when trying to define or understand leadership (Marion and Uhl-Bien 2001; Kellerman 2012; Raffo 2013; Malakyan 2014; Uhl-Bien et al. 2014; Smith-Trudeau 2017; Hanks 2020). Therefore, the leader's success is very much depends upon the attributes of the followers, with Grint (2000, p. 133) adding that followers make the leader and that "it only requires the good follower to do nothing for leadership to fail." As such, understanding followership is vital if leaders are to understand their role and responsibilities as leaders.

It is proposed that leaders cannot function without followers, who act as their eyes and ears and moral compass (in the business world this may even involve customers, and in the health arena must include clients and patients). Leaders cannot achieve much without the "permission" of followers. Leaders often get the praise for the work followers do, and leaders should be aware that much of the credit that rests on their shoulders was first carried on the shoulders of their followers.

Notes On... Nursing Leadership, First Edition. Alison H. James and David Stanley.
© 2024 John Wiley & Sons Ltd. Published 2024 by John Wiley & Sons Ltd.

10.2 Defining Followership

As Crossman and Crossman (2011) point out, definitions of followership are heavily linked to definitions of leadership. More recent words such as "collaborators," "partners," "participants" and even "constituents" are used to describe the changing relationship of followers to leaders (Uhl-Bien 2006). Definitions commonly focus on a dependent leader-follower relationship or a process in which "subordinates" recognise their responsibilities to those in authority or with recognised leadership roles. Most definitions focus on a hierarchical relationship, although a few focus on the interactive nature of the follower–leader relationship (Penny 2017), with followers seen as enthusiastic, active, cooperative and engaged as partners in the leader–follower relationship rather than passive "subordinates" waiting to be told what to do. Carsten et al. (2010, p. 559) view followership as "a role in which followers have the ability to influence leaders and contribute to the improvement and attainment of group and organisational objectives. It is primarily a hierarchically upward influence."

10.3 Follower Responsibilities

Followers' responsibilities are no less important than those of leaders. Follower responsibilities include:

- being active rather than passive (Raffo 2013),
- asking a great deal of the leader, demonstrating respect,
- developing a high degree of literacy about the institution/organisation,
- taking responsibility for achieving their personal and organisational goals, taking ownership of their work,
- connecting themselves to the organisation in meaningful ways,
- becoming loyal to the values of the organisation,
- making a personal commitment and being open to change,
- not blaming a manager or employer for unpopular decisions or policies,
- if they have an opportunity to express an opinion or view, they should do so honestly; "yes men" are poor followers (Wedderburn Tate 1999), and recognise and be aware of their own personal and professional values.

Kellerman (2012) and Malakyan (2014) suggest that in recent years the balance of power has shifted in favour of the followers. Leadership studies and leadership training have commonly neglected the role and place of followers in supporting leadership (Kellerman 2012; Raffo 2013; Malakyan 2014). Even good leaders can be led into making poor decisions and towards ineffective leadership patterns by the actions of empowered and strong followers. Potentially worse, and more often, leaders may be hoodwinked by followers who fool leaders with flattery or hinder them with false realities. The following case is offered as an example of the impact of poor followership. To guard against the influence of ineffective or disruptive followers, leaders need support people who can relay bad news and who can communicate and act on a solid set of values. Leaders also need to encourage open debate and discourse so that they are not protected or insulated from those they lead (Offermann 2005; Penny 2017).

To be effective, followers are required to have the confidence and courage to offer unwelcome advice or information, if required, because leaders require the best and most relevant information if they are to make clear and accurate decisions. Being a follower is not about following, sheep-like, in the wake of a leader because they have authority or because they have been appointed to lead, nor is it about abdicating responsibility and waiting passively for the problems about you to be solved. Followers should be deeply involved in the fabric of an organisation/ward or team and participate by actively engaging with the tasks and duties, decisions and direction under consideration. Effective followership prepares people to be effective leaders (Raffo 2013; Malakyan 2014). Followers should seriously consider questions about their responsibilities to the organisation and leader and be willing to honestly question their capacity to effectively follow before undertaking a followership role. Followers should think about:

- how good are their followership skills?
- are they ready to be engaged as followers?
- are they courageous enough to offer honest and potentially unwelcome information?
- are they ready to change or adapt along the lines the leader is heading?
- are they perceived by their leader as a good follower?
- what style of follower do they present?

Reflective Activity 10.1
Before you read on … Look about your organisation, ward or health-care team. What type of follower are you? What about your fellow followers, what sort of followers are they?

There are several ways to assess the attributes of followers. Kelly (1988) suggested that followers could be identified by five levels of activity and critical thinking. These were sheep/yes people/alienated followers/survivors and effective followers. Douglas (1992) also suggested that followers display a range of followership styles from "very democratic" to "very autocratic." Followership is not easy and can often be inhibited by several factors. These include:

- followers who feel as if they are not "needed" in an organisation or who are undervalued,
- leaders who are not trustworthy,
- leaders who are poor communicators,
- leaders whom the followers find they cannot respect,
- leaders who think followers should read minds (poor communication again),
- poor change processes that exclude followers or neglect their needs or concerns,
- leaders who make poor attempts at getting followers to participate,
- poor attention to rewards (which go far beyond monetary issues),
- leaders who employ inequality, bias, nepotism and unfairness, and
- leaders who are cynical, destructive, hard to approach.

10.4 Good Followers

Good followers do not withhold or avoid difficult options (Varpio and Teunissen 2021). Good followers need to be courageous. They search for other points of view. They seek out the "why" in each situation. They keep the leader honest, give opinions and offer the organisation a chance at greatness. Good followers increase both the leader's chance of getting the job done and the relationships made. Good followers are the keys to leadership success and change. Understanding the needs and concerns of followers is vital for leaders, if they are to engage them in supporting and working effectively together (Varpio and Teunissen 2021).

Looking at the leadership–follower dyad (a group of two) from a post-modern perspective, it might be suggested that it is situational, context-driven or jointly constructed with the leader–follower relationship being almost symbiotic (Malakyan 2014; Varpio and Teunissen 2021). To provide some structure at this point, here are three ways in which the leadership–follower dyad has been construed. Leadership can be explained in terms of a leader–member exchange relationship, where leaders provide direction and support, and followers achieve agreed outcomes. Such approaches define follower characteristics as dependent variables, influenced by a leader (Dvir and Shamir 2003; Penny 2017). The situational leadership theories described follower characteristics as moderator variables (Vroom and Yetton 1973); that is, the characteristics of followers act to influence the relationship between the leader and the follower, and/or the leader and their actions. In general, very little effort has been given to the examination of follower characteristics (as opposed to behaviours) that act as independent variables, that is, follower characteristics that have a direct effect on leader behaviours.

Bass (1990), Ehrhart and Klein (2001), Dvir and Shamir (2003) and Varpio and Teunissen (2021) have each reviewed the relationship of followers to leadership success. Each studied follower behaviour and follower characteristics suggesting that the leaders' success is significantly influenced by the leader–follower relationship. With the following follower characteristics being most beneficial: self-management, team spirit, a positive attitude, a contributor, competent and ethical. Malakyan (2014) and Varpio and Teunissen (2021) are of the view that leadership traits are not superior to followership traits and therefore leadership and followership need to be seen as non-static, dynamic, and leaders and followers need to approach their co-dependence willingly. Effective leadership is an active process that is affected by the characteristics of, and interaction between, the leader, the follower and the context. As such, these variables can be used to both understand these relationships and to better engage as a leader and as a follower. Regardless of the theoretical model involved, it is a discussion about a relationship; that is, it would be reasonable to surmise that a leader–follower dyad works or does not work, depending on the quality or type of relationship bonds (and values-based links) developed between a follower and a leader.

> The best followers have their eyes, ears and minds open. Only fools follow blindly.

10.5 Poor Followers

Not all seemingly compliant followers are "good" or useful. Wedderburn Tate (1999, p. 130) suggested that "*just say yes*" followers support the concept of wanting to please the leader by doing or saying what the leader wants to hear. But she claims that this can lead to the creation of an unhealthy relationship where the yes-sayer and the leader mis-serve each other as the leader is given positive responses by the follower that may misrepresent reality for fear of offending or appearing disloyal. Yes-sayers can be almost sycophantic in their approach to loyalty and rarely offer genuine service to the leader or to the organisation. Leaders may view non-yes-sayers as:

- disloyal,
- causing conflict,
- not telling the truth,
- unwilling to please leaders,
- being troublemakers and
- not being team players.

A leader can recognise and should be on guard for yes-sayers as they tend to:

- monopolise the leader's time,
- offer their views and opinions without being sought,
- be dismissive of comments or feedback by other followers who want to offer realistic information to the leader,
- be dissenting or even bullying of other followers who want to offer realistic feedback to the leader,
- be overprotective of the leader, their vision or values and may be staunchly active (almost fanatical) in defence of the leader if criticised and
- stay "close" to the leader, in personal terms or in proximity; stand by them or sit by them commonly in meetings or at social gatherings.

Followership and leadership are uniquely and inextricably linked by a symbiotic relationship (Wedderburn Tate 1999). Dynamic leadership is dependent on and influenced by the style followers employ and by their capacity to take followership responsibilities seriously. In the same way that effective leaders need to understand and foster their understanding of followership, followers need to recognise they have a responsibility to the leader to be "good" followers. Good followers increase the leader's chance of getting the task or job done; as well they offer an organisation a chance at greatness. In many ways, followers are the key to an organisation and leader's success.

10.6 Summary

Followership is the flip side of leadership and understanding followership is vital for leaders to understand the perspectives of followers. In addition, followers have responsibilities that are at least as important as the leader's responsibilities.

Good followership can be inhibited by poor leadership and leaders should remember that followers are not powerless and good followers have the power to make good leaders better.

References

Abel-Smith, B. (1960) *A History of the Nursing Profession*, London: Heinman.

Ackerman-Anderson, L. & Anderson, D. (2001) *The Change Leader's Roadmap: How to Navigate Your Organization's Transformation*, San Francisco, CA: Pfeiffer.

Adair, J. (1998) *Effective Leadership*, London: Pan.

Algunmeeyn, A., Mrayyan, M.T., Suliman, W.A., Abunab, H.Y. & Al-Rjoub, S. (2023) Effective clinical leadership in hospitals: Barriers from the perspective of nurse managers. *BMJ*. leader-2022-000681. https://doi.org/10.1136/leader-2022-000681. Online ahead of print.

Al-Sabei, S.D., Labrague, L.J., Al-Rawjfah, O., AbuAlRub, R., Burney, I.A. & Jayapal, S.K. (2022) Relationship between interprofessional teamwork and nurses' intent to leave work: The mediating role of job satisfaction and burnout. *Nursing Forum*, 57(4), 568–576. https://doi.org/10.1111/nuf.12706.

Alwazzan, L. (2017) When we say... leadership, we must also say... followership. *Medical Education*, 51, 560.

Andersen, P.O., Jensen, M.K., Lippert, A. & Ostergaard, D. (2010) Identifying non-technical skills and barriers for improvement of teamwork in cardiac arrest teams. *Resuscitation*, 81, 695–702.

Anderson, L. (2012) Difference between nurse leadership vs. management. Nursetogether.com, https://www.nursetogether.com/difference-between-nurse-leadership/ (accessed 22nd June 2023).

Anderson, R.J. (2003) Building hospital–physician relationships through servant leadership. *Frontiers of Health Service Management*, 20(2), 43.

Notes On... Nursing Leadership, First Edition. Alison H. James and David Stanley.
© 2024 John Wiley & Sons Ltd. Published 2024 by John Wiley & Sons Ltd.

Andrews, A., Tierney, S. & Seers, K. (2020) Needing permission: The experience of self-care and self-compassion in nursing: A constructivist grounded theory study. *International Journal of Nursing Studies*, 101, 103436. https://doi.org/10.1016/j.ijnurstu.2019.103436.

Aranzamendez, G., James, D. & Toms, R. (2015) Finding antecedents of psychological safety: A step toward quality improvement. *Nursing Forum*, 50, 171–178. https://doi.org/10.1111/nuf.12084.

Avolio, B.J. & Gardner, W.L. (2005) Authentic leadership development: Getting to the root of positive forms of leadership. *Leadership Quarterly*, 16(3), 315–338.

Babine, R.L., Honess, C., Wierman, H.R. & Hallen, S. (2016) The role of clinical nurse specialists in the implementation and sustainability of a practice change. *Journal of Nursing Management*, 24(1), 39–49. https://doi.org/10.1111/jonm.12269.

Balmer, D.F., Richards, B.F. & Giardino, A.P. (2010) Just be respectful to the primary doc: Teaching mutual respect as a dimension of teamwork in general paediatrics. *Academic Pediatric Association*, 10(6), 372–375.

Banutu-Gomeze, M.B. & Banutu-Gomez, M.T. (2007) Leadership and organizational change in a competitive environment. *Business Renaissance Quarterly*, 2(2), 69.

Bass, B. (2010) *The Bass Handbook of Leadership: Theory, Research, and Managerial Applications*, New York: Simon & Schuster.

Bass, B.M. (1985) *Leadership and Performance Beyond Expectations*, New York: Free Press.

Bass, B.M. (1990) *Bass and Stogdill's Handbook of Leadership: Theory, Research and Management Applications*, New York: Free Press.

Belbin, R.M. (1981) *Management Teams: Why they Succeed or Fail*, Oxford: Butterworth-Heinemann.

Bell, D. & Ritchie, R. (1999) *Towards Effective Subject Leadership in Primary School*, Buckingham: Open University Press.

Bennis, W. & Nanus, B. (1985) *Leaders: The Strategies for Taking Charge*, New York: Harper Row.

Bennis, W., Parikh, J. & Lessem, R. (1995) *Beyond Leadership: Balancing Economics, Ethics and Ecology*, Oxford: Blackwell Business.

Bennis, W.G. (1989) *On Becoming a Leader*, New York: Basic Books.

Bennett, C., James, A. & Kelly, D. (2020) Beyond tropes: Towards a new image of nursing in the wake of COVID-19. *Journal of Clinical Nursing*. http://dx.doi.org/10.1111/jocn.15346.

Bergman, J.Z., Rentsch, J.R., Small, E.E., Davenport, S.W. & Bergman, S.M. (2012) The shared leadership process in decision-making teams. *The Journal of Social Psychology*, 152(1), 17–42.

Berman, A., Frandsen, G., Snyder, S.J., Levett-Jones, T., Burston, A., ... Stanley, D. (2021) *Kozier & Erb's Fundamentals of Nursing* (5th ed.), Sydney, Australia: Pearson.

Bhindi, N. & Duignan, P. (1997) Leadership for a new century: Authenticity, intentionality, spirituality and sensibility. *Educational Management and Administration*, 25(4), 117–132.

Bishop, A. & Smart, T. (1982) (Eds) *Chronicle of Youth: Vera Brittain's war diary 1913 – 1917*. Fontana Paperbacks, Glasgow, Scotland.

Borrill, C., West, M., Shapiro, D. & Rees, A. (2000) Team working and effectiveness in health care. *British Journal of Health Care Management*, 6(8), 364–371.

Bostridge, M. (2008) *Florence Nightingale: The Woman and Her Legend*, London: Penguin/Viking.

Brager, G. & Holloway, S. (1992) *Assessing Prospects for Organizational Change: The Uses of Force Field Analysis*, New York: Haworth Press.

Bresnen, M. (2017) *Managing Modern Healthcare: Knowledge, Networks, and Practice*, Oxfordshire, UK: Routledge. https://doi.org/10.4324/9781315658506.

Brockbank, A. & McGill, I. (2000) *Facilitating Reflective Learning in Higher Education*, Buckingham: Open University Press.

Brown, B. (2016) *Daring Greatly: How the Courage to Be Vulnerable Transforms the Way We Live, Love, Parent, and Lead*, Penguin.

Bruner, J.S. (1986) *Actual Minds, Possible Worlds*, Cambridge, MA: Harvard University Press.

Bryman, A. (1986) *Leadership and Organizations*, London: Routledge.

Budden, L.M., Birks, M., Cant, R., Bagley, T. & Park, T. (2017) Australian nursing students' experience of bullying and/or harassment during clinical placement. *Collegian*, 24(2), 125–133.

Burns, J.M. (1978) *Leadership*, New York: Harper & Row.

Calendrillo, T. (2009) Team building for a healthy work environment. *Nursing Management*, 40(12), 9.

Campbell, P.T. & Rudisill, P.T. (2005) Servant leadership: A critical component for nurse leaders. *Nurse Leader*, 3(3), 27–29.

Cantwell, J. (2015) *Leadership in Action*, Carlton, VA: Melbourne University Press.

Capella, J., Smith, S., Philip, A., Putman, T., Gilbert, C., Fry, R. & Mine, S. (2010) Teamwork training improves the clinical care of trauma patients. *Journal of Surgical Education*, 67(6), 430–443.

Carson, J.B., Tesluk, P.E. & Marrone, J.A. (2007) Shared leadership in teams: An investigation of antecedent conditions and performance. *Academy of Management Journal*, 50(5), 1217–1234.

Carsten, M., Uhl-Bien, M., West, B., Patera, J. & McGregor, R. (2010) Exploring social constructions of followership: A qualitative study. *Leadership Quarterly*, 21, 543–62.

Casey, D. (1993) *Managing Learning Organisations*, Buckingham: Open University Press.

Cherry, R.A., Davis, D.C. & Thorndyke, L. (2010) Transforming culture through physician leadership development. *Physician Executive*, May/June, 38–44.

Christensen, S.S., Wilson, B.L. & Edelman, L.S. (2018) Can I relate? A review and guide for nurse managers in leading generations. *Journal of Nursing Management*, 26(6), 689–695. https://onlinelibrary.com/doi/10.1111/jonm.12601.

Clark, A. & Thompson, D. (2022) Nursing's leadership illusion? Time for more inclusive, credible and clearer conceptions of leadership and leaders. *Journal of Advanced Nursing*, 79(1), e1–e3.

Clark, C.M., Ahten, S.M. & Macey, R. (2013) Using problem-based learning scenarios to prepare nursing students to address incivility. *Clinical Simulation in Nursing*, 9 (3), 75–83. https://doi.org/10.1016/j.ecns.2011.10.003.

Clark, L. (2008) Clinical leadership values beliefs and vision. *Nursing Management*, 15(7), 30–35.

Cline, D., Crenshaw, J.T. & Woods, S. (2022) Nurse leader: A definition for the 21st century. *Nurse Leaders*, August 2022, 381–384.

Cook, M.J. (2001) The renaissance of clinical leadership. *International Nursing Review*, 48(1), 38–46.

Cohen, L. (2015) Anthem, in Berger, J. (ed.), *Leonard Cohen on Leonard Cohen: Interviews and Encounters. Musicians in their own Words*, Chicago Review Press, p. 366, Reprint edition.

Couser, G., Chesak, S. & Cutshall, S. (2020) Developing a course to promote self-care for nurses to address burnout. *OJIN, Online Journal of Issues in Nursing. American Nurses Association*, 25(3).

Coventry, T.H. & Russell, K.P. (2021) The clinical nurse educator as a congruent leader: A mixed method study. *Journal of Nursing Education and Practice*, 11(1), 8–18.

Covey, S.R. (1992) *Principle-Centred Leadership*, London: Simon & Schuster.

Craigie, M., Slatyer, S., Hegney, D., Osseiran-Moisson, R., Gentry, E., Davis, S., Dolan, T. & Rees, C. (2016) A pilot evaluation of a mindful self-care and resiliency (MSCR) intervention for nurses. *Mindfulness*, 7, 764–774.

Crane, P.J. & Ward, S.F. (2016) Self-healing and self-care for nurses. *AORN Journal*, 104(5), 386–400

Creighton, L. & Smart, A. (2022) Professionalism in nursing 2: Working as part of a team. *Nursing Times [online]*, 118, 5.

Crosbie, K. (2006) *Building healthier teams: The impacts of leadership and system practices on the job satisfaction and performance of frontline mental health and addiction workers*, Thesis, Royal Roads University, University of Victoria BC, Canada, November.

Crossman, B. & Crossman, J. (2011) Conceptualising followership – A review of the literature. *Leadership*, 7(4), 481–497.

Curtis, E. & White, P. (2002) Resistance to change. *Nursing Management*, 8(10), 15–20.

Cutcliffe, J. & Cleary, M. (2015) Nursing leadership, missing questions and the elephants in the room: Problematizing the discourse on nursing leadership. *Issues in Mental Health Nursing*, 36, 817–825.

Daft, R.L. (2000) *Management* (5th ed.), Fort Worth, TX: Dryden Press.

Dalai Lama (2000) *The Dalai Lama's Book of Wisdom*, Thorsons Publishers.

Davidson, J.E., Stuck, A.R., Zisook, S. & Proudfoot, J. (2018) Testing a strategy to identify incidence of nurse suicide in the United States. *Journal of Nursing Administration*, 48(5), 259–265.

Dawson, J., West, M. & Yan, X. (2010) Positive and negative effects of team working in healthcare: "real" and "pseudo" teams and their impact on healthcare safety, in Stanton, E., Lemer, C. & Mountford, J. (eds.), *Clinical Leadership: Bridging the Divide*, London: Quay Books.

Day, C., Harris, A., Hadfield, M., Tolley, H. & Beresford, J. (2000) *Leading Schools in Times of Change*, Buckingham: Open University Press.

Deering, S., Johnston, L.C. & Colacchio, K. (2011) Multidisciplinary teamwork and communication training. *Seminars in Perinatology*, 35, 89–96.

de Kok, E., Janssen-Beentjes, J., Lalleman, P., Schoonhoven, L. & Weggelaar, A.M. (2023) Nurse leadership development: A Qualitative Study of the Dutch Excellent Care Program. *Journal of Nursing Management*, Article ID 2368500, 11pp. https://doi.org/10.1155/2023/2368500.

Delaney, M.C. (2018) Caring for the caregivers: Evaluation of the effect of an eight-week pilot mindful self-compassion (MSC) training program on nurses' compassion fatigue and resilience. *PLoS ONE*, 2018(13), e0207261.

Dent, E.R. & Galloway-Goldberg, S. (1999) Challenging resistance to change. *Journal of Applied Behavioural Sciences*, 35(1), 25–41.

Dietz, A., Pronovost, P.J., Menddez-Tellez, P.A., Wyskiel, R., Marsteller, J.A., Thompson. D.A. & Rosen, M.A. (2014) A systematic review of teamwork in the intensive care unit: What do we know about teamwork, team tasks, and improvement strategies. *Journal of Critical Care*, 29, 908–914.

Dignam, D., Duffield, C., Stasa, H., Gray, J., Jackson, D. & Daly, J. (2012) Management and leadership in nursing: An Australian educational perspective. *Journal of Nursing Management*, 20, 65–71.

Dingwall, R., Rafferty, A.M. & Webster, C. (1988) *An Introduction to the Social History of Nursing*, Oxfordshire, UK: Routledge. ISBN 0-415-01786-6.

Douglas, L.M. (1992) *The Effective Nurse Leader and Manager* (4th ed.), St Louis, MO: Mosby.

Drake, K. (2017) The power of networking. *Nursing Management*, 48(9), 56–56. https://doi.org/10.1097/01.NUMA.0000522184.39403.65.

Dublin, R. (1968) *Human Relations in Administration* (2nd ed.), Englewood Cliffs, NJ: Prentice-Hall.

Dubnicki, C. (1991) Building high performance management teams. *Healthcare Forum Journal*, May–June, 1–24.

Duke, D.L. (1986) The aesthetics of leadership. *Educational Administration Quarterly*, 22(1), 7–27.

Dunlap, N.A. (2010) Take your team to the top: Inspire staff to succeed through leadership and motivation. *Journal of Property Management*, 75(1), 28–30.

Dvir, T. & Shamir, B. (2003) Follower developmental characteristics as predicting transformational leadership: A longitudinal field study. *Leadership Quarterly*, 14(3), 327–344.

Dyer, W.G. (1987) *Team Building Issues and Alternatives*, Reading, Massachusetts: Addison Wesley.

Edgehouse, M.A., Edwards, A., Gore, S., Harrison, S. & Zimmerman, J. (2007) Initiating and leading change: A consideration of four new models, *The Catalyst*, 36(2), 3–12.

Egan, G. (1990) *The Skilled Helper: A Systematic Approach to Effective Helping* (4th ed.), Pacific Grove, CA: Brooks/Cole.

Ehrhart, M.G. & Klein, K.J. (2001) Predicting followers' preferences for charismatic leadership: The influence of follower values and personality. *Leadership Quarterly*, 12(2), 153–179.

Eicher-Catt, D. (2005) The myth of servant leadership: A feminist perspective. *Women and Language*, 28(1), 17–26.

Eisenbeiss, S.A., van Knippenberg, D. & Boerner, S. (2008) Transformational leadership and team innovation: Integrating team climate principles. *Journal of Applied Psychology*, 3(6), 1438.

Ellis, P. (2017a) What emotional intelligence is and is not. *WoundsUK*, 13(3), 62–63.

Ellis, P. (2017b) Learning emotional intelligence and what it can do for you. *WoundsUK*, 13(4), 66–68.

Ellis, P. (2021) *Leadership, Management, and Teamworking in Nursing*, London, UK: Learning Matters.

Elloy, D.F. (2008) The relationship between self-leadership behaviours and organizational variables in a self-managed work team environment. *Management Research News*, 31(11), 801–810.

Eslick, M., Wikander, L. & Arnott, N. (2022) Chapter 6: The heart of nursing, in Arnott, N., Paliadelis, P. & Cruickshank, M. (eds.), *The Road to Nursing* (2nd ed.), Cambridge, UK: Cambridge.

Essen, A. & Lindblad, S. (2013) Innovation as emergence in healthcare: Unpacking change from within. *Social Science & Medicine*, 93(September), 203–211.

Falcone, R.A., Daugherty, M., Schweer, L., Patterson, M., Brown, R.L. & Garcia, V.F. (2008) Multidisciplinary pediatric trauma team training using high-fidelity trauma simulation. *Journal of Pediatric Surgery*, 43, 1065–1071.

Fay, B. (1987) *Critical Social Science: Liberation and Its Limits*, Cambridge: Polity Press

Festinger, L. (1957) *A Theory of Cognitive Dissonance*, Stanford, CA: Stanford University Press.

Fiedler, F.E. (1967) *A Theory of Leadership Effectiveness*, New York: McGraw-Hill.

Flusberg, S., Matlock, T. & Thibodeau, P. (2018) War metaphors in public discourse. *Metaphor and Symbol*, 33, 1–18. https://doi.org/10.1080/10926488.2018.1407992.

Foureur, M., Besley, K., Burton, G., Yu, N. & Crisp, J. (2013) Enhancing the resilience of nurses and midwives: Pilot of a mindfulness-based program for increased health, sense of coherence and decreased depression, anxiety, and stress. *Contemporary Nurse*, 2013(45), 114–125.

Francis, R. (2013) *Report of the Mid Staffordshire NHS Foundation Trust Public Inquiry*, London: HM Stationery Office.

Frei, F. & Morriss, A. (2020) Begin with trust: The first step in becoming a genuinely empowering leader, *Harvard Business Review*, 98(3), 112–121. Everything Starts with Trust (hbr.org).

Frendsen, B. (2014) *Nursing Leadership: Management and Leadership Styles, American Association of Nurse Coordination (AANAC)*. www.aanac.org.

Frisch, B. (2008) When teams can't decide. *Harvard Business Review*, 86(11), 121.

Galton, F. (1869) *Hereditary Genius*, New York: Appleton.

George, B. (2003) *Authentic Leadership: Rediscovering the Secrets to Creating Lasting Value*, San Francisco, CA: Jossey-Bass.

Gifford, B.D., Zammuto, R.F., Goodman, E.A. & Hill, K.S. (2002) The relationship between hospital unit culture and nurses' quality of work life. *Journal of Healthcare Management*, 47(1), 13–25.

Goleman, D. (1998a) What makes a leader? *Harvard Business Review*, 76(6), 93–102.

Goleman, D. (1998b) *Working with Emotional Intelligence*, New York: Bantam.

Greenfield, T.B. (1986) Leaders and school: Wilfulness and non-natural order in organizations, in Sergiovanni, T.J. & Corbally, J.E. (eds.), *Leadership and Organizational Culture: New Perspectives on Administration Theory and Practice*, Chicago, IL: University of Chicago Press.

Greenleaf, R.K. (1977) *Servant Leadership: A Journey into the Nature of Legitimate Power and Greatness*, Mahwah, NJ: Paulist Press.

Grenny, J. (2010) Virtual teamwork. *Leadership Excellence*, 27(1), 17.

Griffin, R.W. (1993) *Management* (4th ed.), Boston, MA: Houghton Mifflin.

Grint, K. (2000) *The Arts of Leadership*, Oxford: Oxford University Press.

Grossman, S. & Valiga, T.M. (2021) *The New Leadership Challenge: Creating the Future of Nursing* (5th ed.), Philadelphia, PA: FA Davis.

Guise, J-M. & Segel, S. (2008) Teamwork in obstetric care. *Best Practice and Research in Clinical Obstetrics and Gynaecology*, 22(5), 937–951.

Gumbo, T. (2017) Unpacking the role of leadership and management styles in teaching and research output in South African higher education, Faculty of Engineering and the Built Environment, University of Johannesburg, Johannesburg.

Guttman, H.M. (2008) Leading high performance teams. *Chief Executive*, 231, 33–35.

Handy, C. (1999) *Understanding Organisations* (3rd ed.), London: Penguin.

Hanks, S. (2020) Leadership and followership in a pandemic – Where do you stand? *Journal of the Irish Dental Association*, 66(3), 111.

Hanse, J.J., Harlin, U., Jarebrant, C., Ulin, K. & Winkel, J. (2016) The impact of servant leadership dimensions on leader–member exchange among health care professionals. *Journal of Nursing Management*, 24(2), 228–234. https://doi.org/10.1111/jonm.12304.

Harkins, P. (2008) High-impact team leaders. *Leadership Excellence*, 25(12), 3.

Hart, J. (2010) Team purpose. *Leadership Excellence*, 27(3), 15.

Heinen, M., van Oostveen, C., Peters, J., Vermeulen, H. & Huis, A. (2019) An integrative review of leadership competencies and attributes in advanced nursing practice. *Journal of Advanced Nursing*, 75(11), 2378–2392.

Hendy, J. (2012) The role of the organisational champion in achieving health system change. *Social Science and Medicine*, 74(3), 348–355.

Henriksen, T.D. & Børgesen, K. (2016) Can good leadership be learned through business games. *Human Resource Development International*, 19(5), 388–405. https://doi.org/10.1080/13678868.2016.1203638.

Hersey, P. & Blanchard, K. (1988) *Management of Organisational Behaviour*, Englewood Cliffs, NJ: Prentice-Hall.

Hersey, P., Blanchard, K. & Johnson, D. E. (1996) *Management of Organizational Behaviour: Utilizing Human Resources* (7th ed.), Englewood Cliffs, NJ: Prentice-Hall.

Higgs, J., Cork, S. & Horsfall, D. (2019) *Challenging Future Practice Possibilities*, Leiden, Netherlands: Brill.

Holland, K. (2008) How to build teamwork after an awful session. *New York Times*, late Ed, 8 December, 9.

Hood, K., Cant, R., Baulch, J., Gilbee, A., Leech, M., Anderson, A. & Davies, K. (2014) Prior experience of interprofessional learning enhances undergraduate nursing and healthcare students' professional identity and attitudes to teamwork'. *Nurse Education in Practice*, 14, 117–122.

House, R.J. & Mitchell, T.R. (1974) Path–goal theory of leadership. *Journal of Contemporary Business*, Autumn, 81–97.

Houston, C.J. (2020) *Professional Issues in Nursing: Challenges and Opportunities* (5th ed.), Melbourne, Australia: Wolters Kluwer.

Hurst, K., Ford, J. & Gleeson, C. (2002) Evaluating self-managed integrated community teams. *Journal of Management in Medicine*, 16(6), 463–483.

Hunt, C. & Marini, Z.A. (2012) Incivility in the practice environment: A perspective from clinical nursing teachers. *Nurse Education in Practice*, 12 (6), 366–370. https://doi.org/10.1016/j.nepr.2012.05.001.

Iles, V. (2011a) Why reforming the NHS doesn't work: The importance of understanding how good people offer bad care. March. http://www. reallylearning.com/.

Iles, V. (2011b) Chapter 23: Managing people and teams, *Healthcare Management* (2nd ed.), Maidenhead, Berkshire: Open University Press.

James, A. & Bennett, C. (2020) Effective Nurse Leadership in times of crisis. *Nursing Management*. https://journals.rcni.com/nursing-management/ cpd/effective-nurse-leadership-in-times-of-crisis-nm.2020.e1936/abs, 10.7748/nm. 2020.e1936.

James, A., Bennett, C.L., Blanchard, D. & Stanley, D. (2021a) Nursing and values-based leadership: A literature review, *Journal of Nursing Management*, 1–15. 101111/jonm13273.

James, A.H. (2020) *Perceptions and experiences of leadership: A narrative inquiry of leadership in undergraduate nurse education*, Thesis for Doctor in Advanced Healthcare Practice, Cardiff University Repository, ORCA.

James, A.H., Carrier, J. & Watkins, D. (2021b) Nursing must respond for social justice in this 'perfect storm'. *Editorial. Journal of Advanced Nursing*. https://doi.org/10.1111/jan.14957.

James, A.H. & Arnold, H. (2022) Using coaching and action learning to support staff leadership development. *Nursing Management*. https://doi. org/10.7748/nm.2022.e2040.

James, A.H. & Bennett, C.L. (2022a) Chapter 18: Power, politics and leadership, in Stanley, D., James, A.H. & Bennett, C.L. (eds.), *Clinical Leadership in Nursing and Healthcare* (3rd ed.), London: Wiley, pp. 385–402. https://doi.org/10.1002/9781119869375.ch18.

James, A.H. & Bennett, C.L. (2022b) Chapter 19: From empowerment to emancipation – Developing self leadership, in Stanley, D., James, A.H. & Bennett, C.L. (eds.), *Clinical Leadership in Nursing and Healthcare* (3rd ed.), London: Wiley, pp. 403–420. https://doi. org/10.1002/9781119869375.ch19.

James, A.H., Carrier, J. & Watkins, D. (2022) Perceptions and experiences of leadership in undergraduate nurse education: A narrative inquiry. *Nurse Education Today*. https://doi.org/10.1016/j.nedt.2022.105313.

James, A.H. (2023) Valuing the emotions of leadership learning in nurse education. *Nurse Education in Practice.* https://doi.org/10.1016/j. nepr.2023.103716.

James, A.H., Kelly, D. & Bennett, C.L. (2023) Nursing tropes in turbulent times: Time to rethink nurse leadership? *Journal of Advanced Nursing.* https://doi.org/10.1111/jan.15766.

Jelphs, K. & Dickinson, H. (2008) *Working in Teams (Better Partnership Working)*, Bristol: Policy Press.

Jeong, S.-K. (2018) Concept analysis of teams in nurses, *Journal of Korean Academia-Industrial Cooperation Society*, 19, 482–491.

Jones, L. & Bennett, C.L. (2018) *Leadership in Health and Social Care: An Introduction for Emerging Leaders* (2nd ed.), Banbury: Lantern.

Kaiser, J. (2017) The relationship between leadership style and nurse-to-nurse incivility: Turning the lens inward. *Journal of Nursing Management*, 25, 110–118. https://doi.org/10.1111/jonm.12447.

Kalisch, B.J. & Lee, K.H. (2010) The impact of teamwork on missed nursing care. *Nursing Outlook*, 58, 233–241.

Kalisch, B.J., Lee, K.H. & Rochman, M. (2010) Nursing staff teamwork and job satisfaction. *Journal of Nursing Management*, 198, 938–947.

Kalisch, B.J. & Lee, K.H. (2013) Variations of nursing teamwork by hospital, patient unit, and staff characteristics. *Applied Nursing Research*, 26, 2–9.

Kakabadse, A. & Kakabadse, N. (1999) *Essence of Leadership*, London: International Thomson Business Press.

Katz, R.L. (1955) Skills of an effective administrator. *Harvard Business Review*, 33(1), 33–42.

Kaweckyj, K. (2019) It's all about networking. *The Dental Assistant (1994)*, 88(3), 12–14. f9f9e14f19c44083b9dc87aeffda08d4.pdf.

Kellerman, B. (2012) *The End of Leadership*, HarperCollins, Harvard.

Kelly, D., Horseman, Z., Strachan, F.E., Hamilton, S., Jones, A., Holloway, A., Rafferty, A.M., Noble, H., Reid, J., Harris, R. & Smith, P. (2023) Strengthening the role of the executive nurse director: A qualitative interview study. *Journal of Advanced Nursing.* https://doi.org/10.1111/jan15699.

Kelly, R.E. (1988) In praise of followers. *Harvard Business Review*, 66(6), 142–148.

Kerfoot, K. (2004) The shelf life of leaders. *Medical Surgical Nursing*, 13(5), 348–351.

Kerridge, J. (2013) Why management skills are a priority for nurses. *Nursing Times*, 109(9), 16–17.

Khan, Z.A., Nawaz, A. & Khan, I. (2016) Leadership theories and styles: A literature review. *Journal of Resources Development and Management*, 16, 1–7.

Kim, H.-S. & Sim, I.-O. (2021) The experience of clinical nurses after Korea's enactment of workplace anti-bullying legislation: A phenomenological study. *International Journal of Environmental Research and Public Health*, 18(5711).

Kim, J.-H. (2011) *Resilience*, Goyang: Wisdom House.

Kim, J.S. (2018) *108 Prostrations a Day, 10 Minutes of Miracle to Save my Body*, Seoul: Dawoong, pp. 77–78.

Kim, S.D. (2017) *Let's Transfer the Sutra Coping to Korean Buddhist Practice*, Seoul: Bulkwang Media.

King, C., Edlington, T. & Williams, B. (2020) The 'ideal' clinical supervision environment in nursing and allied health. *Journal of Multidisciplinary Healthcare*, 13, 187–196. https://www.ncbi.nlm.nih.gov/pmc/articles/PMC7034973/.

Kippist, L. & Fitzgerald, A. (2009) Organisational professional conflict and hybrid clinician managers: The effects of dual roles in Australian health care organisations. *Journal of Health Organizations and Management*, 23(6), 642.

Kirkpatrick, S.A. & Locke, E.A. (1991) Leadership: Do traits really matter? *Academy of Management Executive*, 5, 48–60.

Kline, R. (2019) Leadership in the NHS. *BMJ Leader*, 3(4), 129–132.

Kotter, J.P. (1990a) *What leaders really do, Harvard Business Review on Leadership*, Boston, MA: Harvard Business School Press, pp. 37–60.

Kotter, J.P. (1990b) *A Force for Change: How Leadership Differs from Management*, New York: Free Press.

Kotter, J.P. (1996) *Leading Change*, Cambridge, MA: Harvard Business School Press.

Kotter, J.P. (2001) What leaders really do. *Harvard Business Review*, 79(11), 85–96.

Kotterman, J. (2006) Leadership versus management: What's the difference? *The Journal for Quality and Participation*, 29(2), 13–17.

Kouzes, J.M. & Posner, B.Z. (2010) *The Truth about Leadership: The No-fads, Heart of the Matter Facts You Need to Know*, San Francisco: Jossey-Bass.

Kwon, J. (2023) Self-care for nurses who care for others: The effectiveness of meditation as a self-care strategy. *Religions*, 14(1), 90. https://doi.org/10.3390/rel14010090.

LaBrosse, M. (2008) 10 ways to inspire your team. *Corporate Accountant*, 61(3), 58.

Lamothe, M., Boujut, E., Zenasni, F. & Sultan, S. (2014) To be or not to be empathic the combined role of empathic concern and perspective taking in understanding burnout in general practice. *BMC Family Practice*, 15(15).

Lavoie-Tremblay, M., Fernet, C., Lavigne, G.L. & Austin, S. (2015) Transformational and abusing leadership practices: Impacts on novice nurses, quality of care and intention to leave. *Journal of Advanced Nursing*, 73(3), 582–592.

Leanne, S. (2010) *Leadership the Barack Obama Way: Lessons on Teambuilding and Creating a Winning Culture in Challenging Times*, New York: McGraw-Hill.

Leech, D. (2019) Leadership and management are two different roles – what is your job, really? *National Health Executive*. https://www.nationalhealthexecutive.com/Health-Service-Focus/leadership-and-management-are-two-different-roles--what-is-your-job-really (accessed 23rd June 2023).

Leggat, S. (2007) Effective healthcare teams require effective team members: Defining teamwork competencies. *BMC Health Services Research*, 7(17), 1–10.

Leigh, A. & Maynard, M. (1995) *Leading Your Team: How to Involve and Inspire Teams*, London: Nicholas Brealey.

Lencioni, P. (2002) *The Five Dysfunctions of a Team*, San Francisco, CA: Jossey-Bass.

Lessard, L., Morin, D. & Sylvain, H. (2008) Understanding teams and teamwork. *Canadian Nurse*, 104(3), 12–13.

Lett, M. (2002) The concept of clinical leadership. *Contemporary Nurse*, 12(1), 6–20.

Lewin, K. (1951) *Field Theory in Social Science*, New York: Harper & Row.

Lindsay, E. (2018) Importance of attending conferences: Being aware of what is happening around you. *British Journal of Community Nursing*, 23(Sup6), S40–S41. https://doi.org/10.12968/bjcn.2018.23.Sup6.S40.

Litz, B.T., Stein, N., Delaney, E., Lebowitz, L., Nash, W.P., Silva, C. & Maguen, S. (2009) Moral injury and moral repair in war veterans: A pre-liminary model and intervention strategy. *Clinical Psychology Review*, 29, 695–706. https://doi.org/10.1016/j.cpr.2009.07.003.

Lowney, C. (2003) *Heroic Leadership: Best Practices from a 450-Year-Old Company that Changed the World*, Chicago, IL: Loyola Press.

Lyons, V.E. & Popejoy, L.L. (2014) Meta-analysis of surgical safety checklist effects on teamwork, communication, morbidity, mortality and safety. *Western Journal of Nursing Research*, 36(2), 245–261.

MacDonald, C.M., Hancock, P.D., Kennedy, D.M., MacDonald, S.A., Watkins, K.E. & Baldwin, D.D. (2022) Incivility in practice – Incidence and experiences of nursing students in eastern Canada: A descriptive quantitative study. *Nurse Education Today*, 110, 105263.

MacDonald, M.B., Bally, J.M., Ferguson, L.M., Murray, B.L., Fowler-Kerry, S.E. & Anonson, J.M.S. (2010) Knowledge of the professional role of others: A key interprofessional competency. *Nurse Education in Practice*, 10, 238–242.

MacDonald, N. (2010) How to set up a new team. *Estates Gazette*. 7 Aug., *Trade and Industry*, p. 75.

Mahon, M.A., Mee, L., Brett, D. & Dowling, M. (2017) Nurses' perceived stress and compassion following a mindfulness meditation and self-compassion training. *Journal of Research in Nursing*, 2017(22), 572–583.

Malakyan, P.G. (2014) Followership in leadership studies: A case of leader-follower trade approach. *Journal of Leadership Studies*, 7(4), 6–22.

Man, J. (2010) *The Leadership Secrets of Genghis Khan*, London: Bantam.

Mann, R.D. (1959) A review of the relationship between personality and performance in small groups. *Psychological Bulletin*, 56, 402–410.

Mansel, B. & Einion, A. (2019) 'It's the relationship you develop with them': Emotional intelligence in nurse leadership. A qualitative study. *British Journal of Nursing*, 28(21), 1400–1408.

Marion, R. & Uhl-Bien, M. (2001) Leadership in complex organisations. *Leadership Quarterly*, 12, 389–418.

Markiewicz, L. & West, M. (2011) Leading groups and teams, in Swanwick, T. & McKimm, J. (eds), *ABC of Clinical Leadership*, Oxford, UK: Wiley-Blackwell.

Marlow, S.L., Salas, E., Landon, L.B. & Presnell, B. (2016) Eliciting teamwork with game attributes: A systematic review and research agenda. *Computers in Human Behavior*, 55 (part A), 413–423.

Marquis, B.L. & Huston, C.J. (2021) *Leadership Roles and Management Functions in Nursing: Theory and Application* (10th ed.), Melbourne, Australia: Wolters Kluwer Health.

Martin, P. & Snowdon, M. (2020) Can clinical supervision bolster clinical skills and well-being through challenging times? *Journal of Advanced Nursing*, 76, 2781–2782. https://doi.org/10.1111/jan.14483.

Mikaelian, B. & Stanley, D. (2016) Incivility in nursing: From roots to repair. Commentary. *Journal of Nursing Management*, 24(7), 962–969

Melnyk, B.M., Orsoline, L., Tan, A., Arslanian-Engoren, C., Melkus, G., Dunbar-Jacob, J., ... Lewis, L. (2018) A national study links nurses' physical and mental health to medical errors and perceived worksite wellness. *Journal of Occupational and Environmental Medicine*, 60(2), 126–131.

Meterko, M., Mohr, D.C. & Young, G.J. (2004) Teamwork culture and patient satisfaction in hospitals'. *Medical Care*, 42(5), 492–498.

Miles, J.M. & Scott, E.S. (2019) A new leadership development model for nursing education. *Journal of Professional Nursing*, 35(1), 5–11.

Mills, J., Wand, T. & Fraser, F.A. (2015) On self-compassion and self-care in nursing: selfish or essential for compassionate care? *International Journal of Nursing Studies*, 52, 791–793.

Mrayyan, M.T., Algunmeeyn, A., Abunab, H.Y., Kutah, O.A., Alfayoumi, I. & Khait, A.A. (2023) Attributes, skills and actions of clinical leadership in nursing as reported by hospital nurses: A cross-sectional study. *BMJ*. leader-2022-000672, 10.1136/leader-2022-000672.Online ahead of print.

Nene, S.E., Ally, H. & Nkosi, E. (2020) Nurse managers experiences of their leadership roles in a specific mining primary healthcare service in the West Rand. *Curationis*, 43(1), 1–8.

Newhouse, R.P. & Spring, B. (2010). Interdisciplinary evidence-based practice: Moving from silos to Synergy. *Nursing Outlook*, 58, 309–317.

Newman, A., Donohue, R. & Eva, N. (2017) Psychological safety: A systematic review of the literature. *Human Resource Management Review*, 27, 521–535. https://psycnet.apa.org/doi/10.1016/j.hrmr.2017.01.001.

NHS England (2023) https://www.england.nhs.uk/nursingmidwifery/shared-governance-and-collective-leadership/nursing-midwifery-excellence.

NHS Graduate Management Training Scheme (2021) NHS Graduate Management Training Scheme. https://graduates.nhs.uk/ (accessed 23rd June 2023).

NHS Leadership Academy (2021) Healthcare leadership model. https://www.leadershipacademy.nhs.uk/resources/healthcare-leadership-model/ (accessed 23rd June 2023).

Northouse, P.G. (2007) *Leadership: Theory and Practice* (4th ed.), London: Sage.

Offermann, L.R. (2005) When followers become toxic, *Harvard Business Review on the Mind of the Leader*, Boston, MA: Harvard Business School Publishing.

Ockenden Review (2022) Ockenden review: summary of findings, conclusions and essential actions – GOV.UK. www.gov.uk.

Orvik, A., Vagen, S.R., Axelsson, S.B. & Axelsson, R. (2015) Quality, efficiency and integrity: Value squeezes in management of hospital wards. *Journal of Nursing Management*, 23, 65–74.

Ota, M. Lam, L., Gilbert, J. & Hills, D. (2022) Nurse leadership in promoting and supporting civility in health care settings: A scoping review. *Journal of Nursing Management*, 30, 4221–4233.

Parker, G.M. (1990) *Team Players and Teamwork: New Strategies for Developing Successful Collaboration* (2nd ed.), San Francisco: Jossey-Bass.

Pearce, C.L. & Conger, J.A. (2003) *Shared Leadership: Reframing the How's and Why's of Leadership*, Sage.

Pedler, M., Burgoyne, J. & Boydell, T. (2004) *A Manager's Guide to Leadership*, Maidenhead: McGraw-Hill Professional.

Peete, D. (2005) Needed: Servant leaders. *Nursing Homes*, 54(7), 8–10.

Penny, S.M. (2017) Serving, following and leading in health care. *Radiologic Technology*, 88(6), 603–617.

Pettigrew, A.M. & Whipp, R. (1998) *Managing Change for Competitive Success*, Oxford: Blackwell.

Pettigrew, A.M., Woodman, R.W. & Cameron, K.S. (2001) Studying organizational change and development: Challenges for future research. *Academy of Management Journal*, 44(4), 697–713.

Pizzuti, A.G., Patel, K.H., McCreary, E.K., Heil, E., Bland, C.M., Chinaeke, E., Love, B.L. & Bookstaver, P.B. (2020) Healthcare practitioners' views of social media as an educational resource. *PloS One*, 15(2), e0228372-e0228372. https://doi.org/10.1371/journal.pone.0228372.

Pondy, L.R. (1978) Leadership is a language game, in McCall, M.W. Jr & Lombardo, M.M. (eds.), *Leadership: Where Else Can We Go?*, Durham, NC: Duke University Press.

Porter-O'Grady, T. (2017) A response to the question of professional governance versus shared governance. *JONA: The Journal of Nursing Administration*, 47(2), 69–71.

Prado, A.M., Pearson, A.A., Bertelsen, N.S. & Pagán, J.A. (2020) Connecting healthcare professionals in Central America through management and leadership development: A social network analysis. *Globalization and Health*, 16(1), 34–34. https://doi.org/10.1186/s12992-020-00557-4.

Raffo, D.M. (2013) Teaching followership in leadership education. *Journal of Leadership Education*, 12(1), 262–273.

Rashford, N.S. & Coghlan, D. (1994) *The Dynamics of Organisational Levels: A Change Framework for Managers and Consultants*, London: Addison-Wesley.

Rath, T. & Conchie, B. (2008) *Strength based Leadership*, New York: Gallup Press.

Rathert, C. & Fleming, D.A. (2008) Hospital ethical climate and teamwork in acute care: The modelling role of leaders. *Health Care Management Review*, 33(4), 323.

Roberts S.J. (2015) Lateral violence in nursing: A review of the past three decades. *Nursing Science Quarterly*, 28 (1), 36–41.

Robbins, S.P., Millet, B., Cacioppe, R. & Waters-Marsh, T. (2001) *Organisational Behaviour: Leading and Managing in Australia and New Zealand* (3rd ed.), Frenchs Forest, NSW: Prentice Hall.

Robinson, C.A. (2006) The leader within. *Journal of Trauma Nursing*, 13(1), 35–37.

Roh, Y.S., Kim, S.S., Park, S. & Ahn, J-W. (2020) Effects of a simulation with team-based learning on knowledge, team performance, and teamwork for nursing students. *CIN*, 38(7), 367–372

Ross, A., Yang, L., Wehrien, L., Perez, A., Farmer, N. & Bevans, M. (2019) Nurses and health-promoting self-care: Do we practice what we preach? *Journal of Nursing Management*, 27(3), 599–608

Salovey, P. & Mayer, J. (1990) Emotional intelligence. *Imagination, Cognition and Personality*, 9, 185–211.

Sample, J.A. (1984) Nominal group technique: An alternative to brainstorming. *Journal of Extension*, 22(2). https://archives.joe.org/joe/1984march/iw2.php.

Sangvai, D., Lyn, M. & Michener, L. (2008) Defining high-performance teams and physician leadership. *Physician Executive*, Mar/Apr, 44–51.

Sarros, J. & Butchatsky, O. (1996) *Leadership: Australia's Top CEOs Finding Out What Makes Them the Best*, Pymble, NSW: Harper Business.

Seago, J.A. (1996) Culture of troubled work groups. *Journal of Nursing Administration*, 26(9), 41–46.

Scully, N.J. (2015) Leadership in nursing: The importance of recognising inherent values and attributes to secure a positive future for the profession. *Collegian*, 22(4), 439–444.

Shirley, M.R. (2006) Authentic leaders creating healthy work environments for nursing practice. *American Journal of Critical Care*, 15(3), 256–268.

Shortell, S.M., O'Brien, J.L., Carman, J.M., Foster, R.W., Hughes, E.F., Boerstler, H. & O'Connor, E.J. (1995) Assessing the impact of continuous quality improvement/total quality management: Concept versus implementation. *Health Services Research*, 30(2), 377–401.

Siassakos, D., Fox, R., Crofts, J.F., Hunt, L.P., Winter, C. & Draycott, T.J. (2011) The management of a simulated emergency: Better teamwork, better performance. *Resuscitation*, 82, 203–206.

Sist, L., Savadori, S., Grandi, A. Martoni, M., Baiocchi, E., Lombardo, C. & Colombo, L. (2022) Self-care for nurses and midwives: Findings from a scoping review. *Healthcare*, 10, 2473.

Sitzman, K. & Watson, J. (2018) *Caring Science, Mindful Practice: Implementing Watson's Human Caring Theory*, Springer Publishing Company.

Slatyer, S., Craigie, M., Rees, C., Davis, S., Dolan, T. & Hegney, D. (2018) Nurse experience of participation in a mindfulness-based self-care and resiliency intervention. *Mindfulness*, 2018(9), 610–617.

Smama'h, Y., Eshah, N.F., Al-Oweidat, I.A., Rayan, A. & Nashwan, A.J. (2023), The impact of leadership styles of nurse managers on nurses' motivation and turnover intention among Jordanian nurses. *Journal of Healthcare Leadership*, 15, 19–29. https://doi.org/10.2147/JHL.S394601.

Smith, D. (1999) Leadership a hard act to follow. News review. *Sunday Times*. (18th July), p. 6.

Smith-Trudeau, P. (2017) Nursing leadership and followership: Reflections on the importance of followers, *Vermont Nurse Connection*, January, February, March, 2–3.

Spears, L.C. (ed.) (1995) *Reflections on Leadership: How Roberts Greenleaf's Theory of Servant Leadership Influenced Today's Top Management Thinkers*, New York: John Wiley & Sons.

Stanley, D. (2006) Role conflict: Leaders and managers. *Nursing Management*, 13(5), 31–37.

Stanley, D. (2008) Congruent leadership: Values in action. *Journal of Nursing Management*, 64, 84–95.

Stanley, D. (2010) Multigenerational workforce issues and their implications for leadership in nursing. *Journal of Nursing Management*, 18, 846–852.

Stanley, D. & Sherratt, A. (2010) Lamp light on leadership: Clinical leadership and Florence Nightingale. *Journal of Nursing Management*, 18, 115–121.

Stanley, D., Cuthbertson, J. & Latimer, K. (2012) Perceptions of clinical leadership in the St. John Ambulance Service in WA. Paramedics Australasia. *Response*, 39(1), 31–37.

Stanley, D., Latimer, K. & Atkinson, J. (2014) Perceptions of clinical leadership in an Aged Care Residential Facility in Perth, Western Australia. *Health Care Current Reviews*, 2, 122. https://doi.org/10.4172/hccr.1000122.

Stanley, D. (2017a) Congruent Leadership Defined. *JOJ Nursing & Health Care*, 3(3), August 2017.

Stanley, D. (2017b) *Clinical Leadership in Nursing and Healthcare* (2nd ed.), Chichester: Wiley-Blackwell.

Stanley, D., Blanchard, D., Hohol, A., Hutton, M. & McDonald, A. (2017) Health professionals' perceptions of clinical leadership. A pilot study. *Cogent Medicine*, 4(1), 1–7. http://dx.doi.org/10.1080/2331205X.2017.1321193.

Stanley, D. & Stanley, K. (2018) Chapter 15: Being a member of an interprofessional team, in Nick, A., Penny, P. & Mary, C. (eds.), *The Road to Nursing*, pp. 243–255.

Stanley, D. (2019) *Values-Based Leadership in Healthcare: Congruent Leadership Explored*, London: SAGE Publishers. ISBN: 9781526487636.

Stanley, D. & Stanley, K. (2019) Clinical leadership in rural and remote practice: A qualitative study, *Journal of Nursing Management*. https://doi.org/10.1111/jonm12813.

Stanley, D., Bennett C.L. & James, A. (2023) *Clinical Leadership in Nursing and Healthcare*, Oxford: Wiley Blackwell.

Stanton, E. & Chapman, C. (2010). Teamworking and clinical leadership, in Stanton, E., Lemer, C. & Mountford, J. (eds.), *Clinical Leadership: Bridging the Divide*, London: Quay Books.

Stanton, E., Lemer, C. & Mountford, J. (2010) *Clinical Leadership: Bridging the Divide*, London: Quay Books.

Steinemann, S., Berg, B., Skinner, A., DiTullio, A., Anzelon, K., Terada, K.,...Speck, C. (2011) In Situ multidisciplinary, simulation-based teamwork training improves early trauma care. *Journal of Surgical Education*, 68(6), 472–477.

St George, A. (2012) *Royal Navy Way of Leadership*, London: Preface.

Stogdill, R.M. (1948) Personal factors associated with leadership: A survey of the literature. *Journal of Psychology*, 25, 35–71

Stogdill, R.M. (1974) *Handbook of Leadership*, New York: Free Press.

Stoker, J.I. (2007) Effects of team tenure and leadership in self-managing teams. *Personal Review*, 37(5), 564–582.

Strasser, D.C., Smits, S.J., Falconer, J.A., Herrin, J.S. & Bowen, S.E. (2002) The influence of hospital culture on rehabilitation team functioning in VA hospitals, *Journal of Rehabilitation Research and Development*, 39(1), 115–125.

Swanwick, T. & McKimm, J. (2017) *ABC of Clinical Leadership* (2nd ed.), Oxford: Wiley Blackwell.

Swearingen, S. & Liberman, A. (2004) Nursing leadership: Serving those who serve others. *Health Care Manager*, 23(2), 100.

Tannenbaum, R. & Schmidt, W.H. (1958) How to choose a leadership pattern. *Harvard Business Review*, 36, 95–101.

Taylor, G. (2017) Nurse managers: Why emotionally-intelligent leadership matters. *Australian Nursing and Midwifery Journal*, 25(2), 20.

The King's Fund. (2017). Caring to change: how compassionate leadership can stimulate innovation in healthcare. https://www.kingsfund.org.uk/publications/caring-change?gclid=EAIaIQobChMI1eLNj5mM8wIVVqmWCh0KRwKxEAAYASAAEgK1VPD_BwE (accessed 21st June 2023).

Thompson, R. & Kusy M. (2021) Has the COVID pandemic strengthened or Weakened Health Care Teams? A field guide to Healthy Workforce Best Practices. *Nursing Administration Quarterly*, 45(2), 135–141. https://doi.org/10.1097/naq.0000000000000461.

Thorne, M. (2006) What kind of leader are you? *Topics in Emergency Medicine*, 28(2), 104–110.

Towler, A. (2019) Shared leadership, fundamentals benefits and implementation. https://www.ckju.net/en/dossier/shared-leadership-fundamentals-benefits-and-implementation.

Traynor, M. (2017) *Critical Resilience for Nursing*, London: Routledge. https://doi.org/10.4324/9781315638928.

Tuckman, B. (1965) Development sequence in small groups. *Psychology Bulletin*, 63(6), 384–399.

Uhl-Bien, M. (2006) Relational leadership theory: Exploring the social processes of leadership and organising. *Leadership Quarterly*, 17(6), 654–676.

Uhl-Bien, M., Riggio, R.E., Lowe, K.B. & Carson, M.K. (2014) Followership theory: A review and research agenda. *Leadership Quarterly*, 25(1), 83–104.

Valle, Y., Tobias, M.K., Galuska, M.K. & Bailey, K.D. (2022) Three threads for weaving nursing excellence into the fabric of an organization. *Nurse Leader*, 20(1), 20–25.

Varvasovszky, Z. & Brugha, R. (2000) A stakeholder analysis. *Health Policy and Planning*, 15 (3), 338–345. https://doi.org/10.1093/heapol/15.3.338.

Varpio, L. & Teunissen, P. (2021) Leadership in interprofessional healthcare teams: Empowering networking with followership. *Medical Teacher*, 43(1), 32–37.

Veronesi, G., Kirkpatrick, I. & Altanlar, A. (2019) Are public sector managers a "bureaucratic burden"? The case of English public hospitals. *Journal of Public Administration and Research Theory*, 29(2), 193–209.

Vidal-Blanco, G., Oliver, A., Galiana, L. & Sanso, N. (2018) Quality of work life and self-care in nursing staff with high emotional demand. *Enfermeria Clinica*, 29, 186–194. https://www.ckju.net/en/dossier/ shared-leadership-fundamentals-benefits-and-implementation.

Vize, R. (2015) Why doctors don't dare go into management. *The BMJ*, 350(922), 16–18.

Vogelsmeier, A. & Scott-Cawiezell, J. (2009) The role of nursing leadership in successful technology implementation. *Journal of Nursing Administration*, 39(7/8), 313.

Vroom, V. H. & Yetton, P. (1973) *Leadership and Decision Making*, Pittsburgh, PA: University of Pittsburgh Press.

Wageman, R., Fisher, C.& Hackmann, J.R. (2009) Leading teams when the time is right: Finding the best moments to act. *Organizational Dynamics*, 38(3), 192.

Walker, D. (2016) Managing moving pieces. *Talent Management*, November, 42–46.

Walker, T. (2006) Servant leaders. *Managed Healthcare Executive*, 16(3), 20–26.

Watson, C.M. (1983) Leadership, management and the seven keys. *Business Horizons*, 26(2), 8–13.

Wedderburn Tate, C. (1999) *Leadership in Nursing*, London: Churchill Livingstone.

Weihrich, H. & Koontz, H. (1993) *Management at a Global Perspective* (10th ed.), New York: McGraw-Hill.

Weng, R.-H., Huang, C.-Y., Chen, L.-M. & Chang, L.-Y. (2015) Exploring the impact of transformational leadership on nurse innovation behaviour: A cross-sectional study. *Journal of Nursing Management*, 23, 427–439.

West, M. (2021) *Compassionate Leadership: Sustaining Wisdom, Humanity and Presence in Health and Social*, Swirling Leaf Press.

West, M., Armit, K., Loewenthal, L., Eckert, R., West, T. & Lee, A. (2015) *Leadership and Leadership Development in Health Care: The Evidence Base*, London: Faculty of Medical Leadership and Management/King's Fund/Center for Creative Leadership. http://www.kingsfund.org.uk/ sites/files/kf/field/field_publication_file/leadership-leadership-development-health-care-feb-2015.pdf (accessed 17th June 2023).

West, M., Eckert, R., Collins, B. & Chowla, R. (2017) *Caring to change: How compassionate leadership can stimulate innovation in health care*, The Kings Fund, May, 1–39.

Wilson, J.L. (2016) An exploration of bullying behaviours in nursing: A review of the literature, *British Journal of Nursing*, 25(6), 340. https://doi. org/10.12968/bjon.2016.25.6.303.

Wood, C. (2021) Leadership and management for nurses working at an advanced level, *British Journal of Nursing*, 30(5), 282–286.

Wong, C. & Cummings, G. (2009) Authentic leadership: A new theory for nursing or back to basics?, *Journal of Health Organisations and Management*, 23(50), 522.

World Health Organization. (1988) *Learning Together to Work Together for Health. Report of a WHO Study Group on Multi-Professional Education of Health Personnel: The Team Approach*, Geneva: WHO, p. 769.

World Health Organization (WHO). (2022) *Guidelines of Self-care Interventions for Health and Wellbeing*, Geneva, Switzerland: World Health Organisation.

Worline, M.C. & Dutton, J.E. (2017) *Awakening Compassion at Work: The Quiet Power that Elevates People and Organizations*, Berrett-Koehler Publishers.

Wynendaele, H., Gemmel, P., Pattyn, E., Myny, D. & Trybou, J. (2021) Systematic review: What is the impact of self-scheduling on the patient, nurse and organization? *Journal of Advanced Nursing*, 77, 47–82.

Yoder-Wise, P.S. (2015) *Leading and Managing in Nursing* (6th ed.), London: Mosby

Zaccaro, S.J., Rittman, A.L. & Marks, M.A. (2001) Team leadership, *Leadership Quarterly*, 12, 451–483.

Zaleznik, A. (1977) *Managers and leaders: Are they different? Harvard Business Review on Leadership*, Boston, MA: Harvard Business School Press, pp. 61–88.

Web References

Florence Nightingale quote: (accessed 20th June 2023). https://www.azquotes.com/quote/614045.

Leadership definition NODE 2021: (accessed 21st June 2023). https://www.tlu.ee/~sirvir/Leadership/The%20Concept%20of%20Leadership/definitions_of_leadership.html#:~:text=Conclusion-,Definitions%20of%20Leadership,'%20(NODE%2C%202001).

Marie Morganelli article with the Bell (2021) quote: (accessed 27th June 2023) https://www.snhu.edu/about-us/newsroom/health/what-is-nurse-leadership#:~:text=Nurse%20leadership%20is%20the%20ability,Dr.

The Social Dilemma (accessed 17th June 2023).

https://www.amnesty.org.au/the-social-dilemma-2/?cn=trd&mc=click&pli =23501504&PluID=0&ord={timestamp}&gclid=EAIaIQobChMIqKumu sjL_wIVaZhmAh2lOAZMEAAYAyAAEgKew_D_BwE).

Privacy and the Internet (accessed 4th June 2023).

https://www.amnesty.org/en/documents/pol30/1404/2019/en/.

The Bounce Back Project (accessed 18th June 2023).

https://www.feelinggoodmn.org/what-we-do/bounce-back-project-/5-pillars-of-resilience/#:~:text=Resilience%20is%20made%20up%20of, Care%2C%20Positive%20Relationships%20and%20Purpose.

Jenna Liphart Nurse Together: 5 Leadership attributes (accessed 27th June 2023).

https://www.nursetogether.com/5-leadership-qualities-every-nurse-should-have/.

Mind Tools (2023) (SWOT Analysis) (accessed 27th June 2023).

https://www.mindtools.com/amtbj63/swot-analysis.

Mind Tools 2023 (PEST Analysis) (accessed 27th June 2023).

https://www.mindtools.com/aqa3q37/pest-analysis.

Indeed.com (6 benefits of teamwork in nursing and ways to improve it). (accessed 29th June 2023).

https://ca.indeed.com/career-advice/career-development/teamwork-in-nursing.

Vulnerability quotes by Brené Brown (2016) (accessed 7th September 2023).

https://www.happierhuman.com/brene-brown-quotes/#:~:text=%E2%80%9CVulnerability%20is%20the%20birthplace%20of,%2C%20vulnerability%20is%20the%20path.%E2%80%9D

Theodore Roosevelt - Quote, "Man in the Arena" (1910) (accessed 7th September 2023).

https://buchilly.medium.com/the-man-in-the-arena-a52098b31d2e.

Index

Notes On... Nursing Leadership, First Edition. Alison H. James and David Stanley.
© 2024 John Wiley & Sons, Ltd. Published 2024 by John Wiley & Sons, Ltd.